The Guide to Mental Health for Nurses in Primary Care

Edited by
Elizabeth Armstrong

Forewords by

Jackie Carnell
and
Godfrey Mazhindu

Radcliffe Medical Press

Radcliffe Medical Press Ltd
18 Marcham Road
Abingdon
Oxon OX14 1AA
United Kingdom

www.radcliffe-oxford.com
The Radcliffe Medical Press electronic catalogue and online ordering facility.
Direct sales to anywhere in the world.

_____

British Library Cataloguing in Publication Data

A catalogue record for this book is available from the British Library.

ISBN 1 85775 435 2

Typeset by Aarontype Ltd, Easton, Bristol
Printed and bound TJ International Ltd, Padstow, Cornwall

Contents

Foreword

Much of Liz Armstrong's professional life has been driven by the desire to see mental health taken seriously and viewed as a priority within primary care. This book could do much to make this a reality. In her own words, 'Mental health is part of healthcare, not an optional extra'.

The following chapters will convince primary care nurses that they are not an 'optional extra' to the care and treatment of people in the community suffering from, or prone to, mental illness. It will provide them with the knowledge, confidence and motivation to become key players alongside GP colleagues and acute services.

The Mental Health National Service Framework is more than just another policy document. It is also the vehicle that has the potential to make a real difference to people's lives by recognising that their feelings matter; that feeling good should not be another 'optional extra'. Ninety out of every 100 people suffering from mental illness will receive treatment solely from within primary care. These chapters should help primary care teams to meet their responsibilities in meeting the first three standards within the framework.

I was so pleased that this book highlights the importance of the right environment for care to be given. Dismal, dreary and inconvenient premises do not inspire confidence and hope in already depressed people. We have always underestimated the effect of the environment on both service users and providers.

I was also pleased to see the importance placed on the morale and well being of the primary care staff themselves. Stressed and tired staff, who do not feel valued members of the team, cannot rise to the challenges outlined here.

This book can provide a valuable resource and inspiration to all primary healthcare team members, not just the health professionals within it. It will provide them not only with knowledge, but also with a shared sense of purpose to plan and deliver a real team approach to mental health. The sum of the whole is always greater than the sum of all its parts.

Above all, it gives a sensible and balanced recognition to the vital contribution that all primary care nurses employed by, or attached to, the practice make to the mental health needs within their population.

Jackie Carnell
Director
Community Practitioners' and Health Visitors' Association
October 2001

Foreword

Over the past few years, the UK Government has published a number of Consultation Documents, Health Service Circulars (HSC) and Policy Directives on the subject of Mental Health and Mental Health Care. Numerous academic and professional articles and books have also been written, covering a wide range of related aspects, including access to services, diagnosis and treatment.

Recent years have witnessed a shift in emphasis from long-term institutional and acute hospital care to community care for people who experience mental health problems. The focus of care increasingly embraces health promotion and prevention, and places particular responsibility on service users in relation to self-care and the support, care and treatment provided by carers and community-based professional and support staff, particularly GPs, nurses and other health and social care professionals. Equally, the relationship between mental health and psychosomatic physical symptoms has been widely reported. In this context, there is some evidence to suggest that early detection, management and treatment of both diagnosed and unrecognised mental health problems is an important cost reduction measure, as reflected in the corresponding reduction in unnecessary referrals for physical investigation and treatment. The combined effect of these developments suggests there is a need to develop and enhance the coping strategies of service users, provide information and support for carers, and reform the preparation of practitioners in a manner that takes account of new and emerging imperatives.

Evidence available from the literature suggests that many of the current texts on primary care mental health have been written by doctors, and generally reflect a medical perspective. Consequently, texts that are accessible to the wider frontline professional workforce within community health and social care settings are to be welcomed.

This book is written by and for nurses. It contains practical ideas and is not loaded with philosophical and theoretical concepts and jargon, but is written in a style that also makes it accessible to the wider health and social care workforce, carers and service users. The arguments presented in each chapter are based on published evidence and the authors also make effective use of their collective experience and that of significant others engaged in this field. The book reflects an up-to-date position and is challenging and realistic. It also adopts a pro-active stance that breaks new ground – its publication is timely.

Professor Godfrey Mazhindu
Director of the Centre for Healthcare Education
University College Northampton
October 2001

List of contributors

Elizabeth Armstrong
Executive Director
Depression Care Training Centre
University College, Northampton
Trustee, PriMHE

Jim Barnard
Primary Care Adviser
Substance Misuse Advisory Service (SMAS)
London

Martin Davies
Mental Health Trainer
Depression Care Training Centre
University College, Northampton

Bev Hallpike
Community Mental Health Team Leader for Older People
Daventry

Ann Mitchell
Undergraduate Framework Co-ordinator
Centre for Health Care Education
University College, Northampton

Simon Morton
Primary Care Adviser
Substance Misuse Advisory Service (SMAS)
London

Heather Raistrick
Mental Health Lead
Development Manager
Bradford South and West Primary Care Trust

Sheelah Seeley
Research Assistant
University of Reading

Acknowledgements

I should like to thank the following friends and colleagues for their contributions to this book and for providing me with helpful suggestions and ideas. Primarily, Tony Ryan, whose idea the book was and who had intended to write it with me, but unfortunately had to withdraw because of a family tragedy. I hope he will feel that we have not let him down. Sheelah Seeley's help with Chapter 1 was invaluable, especially much useful discussion on postnatal mental illness.

Martin Davies, who co-wrote Chapter 2 and contributed Chapter 3, has been an inspirational colleague at the Depression Care Training Centre over several years. His help and support have been much appreciated. Jim Barnard and Simon Morton coped with Chapter 4 in spite of the rather short notice. Heather Raistrick managed to help with Chapter 6 whilst also doing her dissertation. Bev Hallpike took up the challenge of Chapter 7 even though she had not done anything like it before. Ann Mitchell's insights in Chapter 8 have given me new food for thought, and she kindly offered to read an early draft of the manuscript, for which I am very grateful.

Sally Gardner and Joan Foster have contributed valuable information from their pioneering work; Sally as a practice nurse who cares for people with depression in the practice where she works, and Joan who founded and leads the Association of Counsellors in Primary Care. Mike Scanlan read, and made valuable suggestions on, the final manuscript.

Many other friends and colleagues have contributed to my knowledge and experience in this field over the years. Without them, writing this book would not have been possible.

I am aware that I gave my contributors quite a challenge to produce a practical, accessible text for general nurses, for whom mental health is only one of the issues with which they have to contend. Only our readers will tell us how far we have succeeded.

Liz Armstrong
October 2001

Introduction

The National Service Framework for Mental Health was published by the Government towards the end of 1999.[1] The framework is intended to provide a new vision for the care of people with mental health problems in England, and focuses on adults of working age. It highlights the importance of the role of primary care in mental health, acknowledging that most people with mental health problems are cared for by primary care teams alone. Out of every one hundred people who consult their GP with a mental health problem, only about nine will be referred to specialist mental health services. The National Service Framework was designed to improve mental health care over all, not simply to improve specialist services!

The Framework contains seven standards:

- Standard 1 – Mental health promotion
- Standards 2 and 3 – Primary care and access to services
- Standards 4 and 5 – Effective services for people with severe mental illness
- Standard 6 – Caring about carers
- Standard 7 – Preventing suicide.

For Standards 2 and 3, primary care organisations are intended to be the lead agency for implementation. They are key partners in all the other standards. However, it is clear that, if primary care organisations implement the standards for which they are intended to take the lead, they will in fact meet most of their obligations under the other standards. Taking the lead means being pro-active, not waiting for others to tell you what to do.

This presents a challenge to primary care groups, trusts and the GP practices within them. It presents the challenge, not just to the managers and board members, but to every GP and primary care nurse.

This book is partly designed to help primary care nurses rise to the challenge and play their part in implementing the National Service Framework standards. But it is not about writing protocols and guidelines that sit on shelves unread, unused and never implemented. Primarily, this is a practical book. The National Service Framework is about 'driving up the quality of care'. This book is about the practical things that nurses can do to improve the care of people with mental health problems in their place of work.

Common mental disorders have been shown to cause levels of disability similar to those associated with respiratory and cardiovascular disorders.[2] Moreover, there is some evidence that when patients with 'hidden' or unrecognised mental health problems are recognised and treated, health expenditure may be reduced. This is often because of a reduction in referrals for unnecessary physical investigations.[3]

Primary care teams see the full range of people with mental health problems, from those who are distressed but have few symptoms to those with severe illness. Nurses as well as doctors come into contact with many of these people. Often, particularly for people with mild depression or anxiety symptoms, primary care nurses may be able to offer appropriate help without necessarily having to refer either to a GP or to a community mental health nurse. The problem for many nurses is to identify those who need referral and also to have sufficient skills and tools to be able to help the others.

The writers of this book have tried to tackle these issues head on. We have tried to do this in an accessible way, rather than being overly academic. Where the evidence for a particular intervention exists, we have quoted it, but we have not been frightened of using experience either. The research base for primary care mental health is improving, but there is still a need for much more, particularly in nursing. We have recognised too, that most nurses working in primary care are generalists, with generalist roles. The mental health issues their patients and clients bring are only part of the picture, albeit an important and often neglected part. We also appreciate the pressures that nurses, as well as doctors, are under in primary care settings. Time is always in short supply. The key is to use the time you have to the patient's best advantage.

The basis of the diagnostic criteria and clinical guidelines we have used is, where possible, the *World Health Organization's Guide to Mental Health in Primary Care* (UK version).[4] This is based on the primary care version of the 10th edition of the International Classification of Diseases (ICD-10 PHC). The UK version was published in 2000 after extensive consultation and testing. The final version was put together by a national consensus group of a wide range of professionals, including nurses. The full reference details for the WHO Guide are given below. They will not be repeated in each chapter.

There are other books on primary care mental health, but most have been written by doctors from a medical standpoint. This is a book for nurses, celebrating the nursing contribution to primary mental health care.

References

1 Department of Health (1999) *National Service Framework for Mental Health: modern standards and service models.* Department of Health, London.

2 Murray CJL and Lopez AD (eds) (1996) *The Global Burden of Disease: a comprehensive assessment of mortality and disability from diseases, injuries and risk factors in 1990 and projected to 2020.* Published by the Harvard School of Public Health on behalf of the World Health Organization and the World Bank.

3 Morriss R, Gask L, Ronalds C *et al.*(1998) Cost effectiveness of a new treatment of somatised mental disorder taught to GPs. *Family Practice.* **1**5(2): 119–25.

4 WHO (2000) *WHO Guide to Mental Health in Primary Care* (UK Version). Royal Society of Medicine, London. www.whoguidemhpcuk.org.

CHAPTER ONE

Depression

Elizabeth Armstrong and Sheelah Seeley

Introduction

Depression is the most common mental illness encountered in primary care settings. As a chronic illness, it is more common than either asthma or diabetes, yet people with depression still struggle for the recognition and treatment that this debilitating condition demands. Depression not only affects the sufferer directly but also has serious consequences for family relationships, work and social life.

The good news about depression is that it is treatable. Furthermore, there is a great deal that nurses can do to help patients and clients with depressive illness. People with fewer symptoms who do not require medical treatment can often be cared for by nurses alone. For those with more severe illness, effective care may be provided by a nurse in collaboration with the doctor. There are also possibilities for collaboration between primary care nurses and counsellors or community mental health nurses. Such collaboration is not yet as widespread as it ought to be.

The diagnosis of depression

The key feature of depression is a lowering of mood. Everyone feels low from time to time and many people may describe themselves as being 'depressed', but for this low mood to reach the level at which it can be described as an illness, certain criteria must be met.

The *WHO Guide to Mental Health in Primary Care* (2000) lists the diagnostic features as:

- low or sad mood
- loss of interest or pleasure

with at least four of the following associated symptoms:

- disturbed sleep*
- disturbed appetite*
- guilt or low self-worth*
- pessimism or hopelessness about the future
- decreased libido
- diurnal mood variation
- poor concentration*
- suicidal thoughts or acts*
- loss of self-confidence
- fatigue or loss of energy*
- agitation or slowing of movement or speech.*

Symptoms of anxiety or nervousness are also often present. If low mood and loss of interest have been present for more than two weeks and four or more of the symptoms marked * are present, this is a severe depressive illness and such patients will need to be considered for medication.

   Some physical illnesses, such as parkinsonism, multiple sclerosis and hypothyroidism, produce depressive symptoms as do some drugs, for example, betablockers, other antihypertensives, H2 blockers, oral contraceptives and corticosteroids. These conditions should be excluded before the diagnosis of depression is made.

Types of depression

There have been many ways of classifying depression over the years, some of which are less useful than others. In practice it is often most helpful to see depression in terms of a continuum from the normal low mood which everyone can experience from time to time through to mild, moderate and severe symptom levels.[1] This 'depression continuum' can be used to explain to patients what depression is and also to demonstrate that, at the moderate to severe level, medical treatment may be required.

The Depression Continuum

Normal   *Mild*   *Moderate*   *Severe*

Other classifications commonly encountered are as follows.

Reactive or endogenous

'Reactive' depression is said to be that which occurs in response to a major life event. 'Endogenous' depression is said to arise spontaneously without an obvious trigger. This classification is now considered rather old-fashioned. It has dangers because it may lead to a belief that reactive depression does not require treatment. In fact most experts would say that an illness which reaches the criteria above will require treatment whatever the supposed cause.

Bipolar or unipolar

Bipolar depression (also known as manic depression or manic depressive psychosis) involves mood swings between severe depression and high elation (*see* Chapter 6). Unipolar depression is depression without the accompanying mood swings. The latter is the most common type of depression, but there are overlaps between the two. Bipolar depression is strongly familial, unipolar depression is less so.

Neurotic or psychotic

In this context, the word 'neurotic' does not mean that the patient is an attention-seeking nuisance. It simply means 'mood disorder' without psychotic features such as delusions or hallucinations. Psychotic features may be present in more severe episodes of depression. Psychotic symptoms always indicate the need for referral to psychiatric services. Neurotic depression may also be referred to as 'non-psychotic' depression.

Dysthymia

This is also a term in common use. It describes a chronic lowering of mood which may last for several years. It may not reach the criteria for severe depression and sufferers may continue to function but relationships may be affected. There may be acute exacerbations.

Postnatal depression

There are three types of postnatal psychological disturbance: the 'blues', depression and psychosis. The 'blues' affects about 50–70% of mothers. It is usually mild with maybe a day or two of transient tearfulness in the first ten days after childbirth, but it may go on to develop into a depressive episode.

Postnatal depression is an illness, essentially identical to depression at any other time, with the added complication of the usual demands of caring for a baby. It affects about 10–15% of women in the year following childbirth, the majority of onsets occurring during the first one to three months. It is not uncommon for fathers to suffer depression at this time. Depression is almost as common in pregnancy as it is afterwards, although it is not always the case that one follows or precedes the other.

About two in 1000 women will develop psychotic illness within four weeks of childbirth (also called puerperal psychosis). This is a severe disorder characterised by symptoms such as hallucinations, delusions and gross impairment of functioning. The onset is rapid and dramatic, requiring inpatient treatment with the baby if possible. With prompt treatment the prognosis is normally good. Women with a personal or family risk of bipolar disorder have a higher risk of developing this condition (*see* Chapter 6).

There is also an increasing body of evidence to suggest that post-traumatic stress disorder (*see* Chapter 2) may occur following childbirth where the experience has been particularly distressing.[2]

Seasonal affective disorder (SAD)

This is depression which occurs during the darker winter months, often recurring year after year. Some researchers believe that the hormone, melatonin, plays a part in the disorder since there appears to be a seasonal variation in levels of the hormone. There may also be a variation in hormone levels during dark hours and daylight.[3] Many people with the condition find light therapy helpful. Seasonal variations in symptoms may occur in other forms of depressive illness.

Chronic fatigue syndrome

This syndrome, which may also be known as 'ME', is characterised by extreme tiredness after both mental exertion and little physical effort. It may follow a viral infection, trauma or other physical illness. Depressive symptoms may be present, but will not usually reach the criteria for severe depression. However, people with chronic fatigue syndrome may become depressed because of the debilitating effects of the illness – as is the case with any other chronic illness.[4]

Causes of depression

Depression is a complex illness with no single cause. There have been a number of theories trying to explain how the condition develops, but no individual explanation seems to satisfy all situations.

Genetics

Heredity plays a part, especially in bipolar depression which is more common in first degree relatives of sufferers than in the general population. It seems possible that some people may inherit a tendency to depression. The illness may then be triggered by other factors.[4]

Biochemistry

Brain chemistry is also involved in depression. Changes in both the stress mechanisms and in the neurotransmitters have been identified. The neurotransmitters serotonin and noradrenaline have been particularly studied. Levels are lowered in depressive illnesses. Most antidepressants are designed to act on this system, raising serotonin and/or noradrenaline levels. The biochemical changes take time to develop and to be corrected and this explains why antidepressants take time to have their effect. It is still unclear whether it is the low level of neurotransmitters that causes depression or whether depression causes the level to drop. As yet there is no blood test to diagnose depression.

   Depression is linked with alcohol misuse. People with depression may use alcohol in an attempt to obtain relief or escape from their symptoms. Alcohol is a central nervous system depressant and is likely to make existing depression worse, quite apart from the damage it may do to family and social relationships. Excessive drinking is well recognised as a physical health risk. Its effect on mental health is just as serious.

Psychology

A variety of psychological explanations for depression have been proposed. In psycho-analytical theory it was held that depression was caused by loss, particularly loss which involved a threat to self. Cognitive theory, which underlies the principles of cognitive behavioural therapy, suggests that people who suffer from depression have a characteristic negative view of self, the world and the future.[5] Learning theory cites 'learned helplessness' as significant. In this set of ideas, the person who is vulnerable to depression is the person who has learned to feel that they have no control over what happens to them.[3]

Risk factors

A useful way of thinking about depression may be to see it in terms of three sets of factors.

- Predisposing factors which increase vulnerability.
- Precipitating factors which trigger the illness.
- Maintaining factors which keep the illness going and prevent recovery.

Each factor has biological, social and psychological components.[6]

Predisposing factors include:

- *biological*: genetic (especially bipolar disorder); physical deprivation in childhood
- *social*: emotional deprivation in childhood; bereavement; chronic work or marital problems; lack of personal and social support

- *psychological*: poor parental role models; low self-esteem; 'learned help-lessness'.

Precipitating factors include:

- *biological*: recent infections; disabling injury; malignant disease or other life-threatening illness
- *social*: recent loss or threat of loss, e.g. bereavement, loss of job or threat of redundancy or loss of a supporting relationship
- *psychological*: inappropriate or maladaptive responses to loss leading to feelings of helplessness or hopelessness.

Maintaining factors include:

- *biological*: chronic pain and disability, especially hearing loss or sight impairment, both of which predispose to social isolation
- *social*: chronic problems with housing, finance, work, marriage, family and/or friends; lack of an intimate, confiding relationship at home; lack of practical help and information about how to deal with social difficulties
- *psychological*: low self-esteem; doubts about personal recovery from illness; the effects of long-term dependency on benefits.

Even though depressive symptoms are common during bereavement, most bereaved people do not suffer a clinical depressive illness. Bereavement is a normal process involving periods of intense sadness. It may, however, sometimes trigger a depressive illness which, in turn, may require treatment. This is particularly the case when the bereavement process is complicated by other factors such as chronic social difficulties and a previously ambivalent relationship with the deceased.[7] Most people who have suffered loss do not require antidepressant treatment, but they may well benefit from an explanation of the grieving process. These days, many people may reach middle age without ever having experienced the loss of a loved one. The grieving process is not as well understood by ordinary people as it was in the past, and rituals of mourning are not so socially acceptable.

In postnatal depression there is a widely held belief that hormones have a part to play. Evidence suggests that the 'blues' and puerperal psychosis, with their early postnatal onset, do have a relationship with hormone levels.[8] The evidence for a biological basis for postnatal depression is equivocal. Social and psychological risk factors may be more significant, so that the absence of social and marital support, and a previous history of depression are very important. Sheppard (1997) has reported a study of women consulting health visitors in both urban and rural areas.[9] He found that depression was significantly related to social and economic disadvantage, family disruption and family size, and suggests that what he calls 'poor life chances' lie behind much of the data.

Older people are vulnerable to depression, with studies estimating that up to 15% of people over 65 may be depressed. However, this still means that most older people do not become depressed and that depression is not a natural consequence of being old. Depression in older people is as treatable as it is at any other age, by psychological methods as well as by medication. Confusion or apparent cognitive impairment may be present in elderly people with depression. Thus, there is a danger of misdiagnosing depression as dementia (*see* Chapter 7).

Depression occurs in children and in adolescents. The way children react to distress will vary according to their age and stage of development. For example, a young child may exhibit behavioural problems whereas an older teenager may show symptoms very like adult depression. Depression in children needs to be understood in the context of the family and there may be links with child abuse, especially sexual abuse.[4] Practice nurses report that it is not uncommon to find adult women with depression disclosing previous sexual abuse during childhood. Childhood depression is rarely treated using drugs. Family approaches are likely to be more beneficial.

Recognition of depression

The ability of professionals to recognise depression in their patients and clients varies widely. Most people with depressive illnesses do not go to their doctor and immediately say they are depressed. They may present with a variety of symptoms, often physical, such as pain or feeling 'tired all the time'. They may be anxious or unable to sleep or be worried about social difficulties such as financial problems or problems with relationships.

Doctors who are good at recognising depression show interest and concern, ask about home, work and family and make use of the verbal and non-verbal cues which patients give.[10] They also have good interviewing skills such as making more eye contact, listening without interruption, asking open-ended questions, asking about feelings and making empathic comments.

Patients in whom the illness is recognised are more likely to be white, female, middle-aged, unemployed, bereaved or separated and to look depressed. The illness is less likely to be recognised in adolescents, young adults, older people, students, people with physical illness or people who present with physical symptoms. Difficulties in recognition may appear if patients are reluctant to consider psychological problems or if psychological cues are given late in the interview or not at all.

Interviewing skills are important for nurses as well as doctors. Part of the nurse's role in the consultation may be to facilitate access to the doctor.[11] To do this effectively for a person with depression, the nurse will need to be able to list the patient's symptoms and to help the patient understand that some of their unexplained symptoms might be due to depression and that depression is a treatable illness.

Assessment of depression

The first step in assessment is to be able to recognise those people who are suffering from severe depression because these are the people who are most likely to respond to antidepressant therapy. There is no evidence that people with mild depressive symptoms will benefit from medication. Many people with mild depression will recover spontaneously.

That is not to say that people with mild to moderate depression do not require help, but there are a variety of ways of offering help which do not involve medication (*see* Chapter 3). There is evidence to suggest that in postnatal depression, mild to moderate conditions may be of particular importance. Depressive symptoms at these levels interfere with the normal communications between mother and baby in the early months. In a significant number of cases the resultant difficulties in the mother/baby relationship have adverse effects on the child's cognitive, emotional and behavioural development.[12]

Thus, it is important for a nurse to become familiar with the list of symptoms of depression, and a method of eliciting them in a systematic way so that appropriate referrals can be made to the GP.

A useful screening question which can be used at any time is simply to ask a patient or client 'How are you feeling in yourself?' Any answer which indicates a possible low mood can then be followed up with further questions about symptoms. Of course, there is no need to use follow-up questions with a person who is not experiencing a low mood.

Where low mood is present, questions then need to be specifically about symptoms, for example:

- Have you lost interest in things?
- Are you feeling more tired than usual?
- Have you lost confidence in yourself?
- How are you sleeping?
- How is your appetite? Is it different from usual? Have you lost/gained weight?
- Do you feel guilty about things?
- Are you finding it difficult to concentrate?
- Do you feel that life is not worth living any more?

When assessing symptom level, asking direct questions such as these is important. Not only does it help the nurse decide how severe the patient's problem is but it may also help the patient to understand what is happening to them. The realisation that they are suffering from an illness and not 'going mad' may be the first step towards accepting treatment and recovering.

Other aspects which need to be assessed include:

- social network (availability of a confidante; someone to talk to)
- view of self – self-esteem
- past history – personal and family
- biological symptoms, for example backache or headaches.

Assessment in postnatal depression may present particular difficulties in that some mothers may believe that their baby will be taken away from them if they admit to psychological difficulties, particularly if these include negative feelings about the baby. Mothers may need reassurance that modern practice is to do everything possible to support the mother to enable her to care for her baby at home. Most health visitors try to deal with this problem by addressing issues of postnatal depression from the beginning. An assessment would start from the assumption that this is a special time for mother and baby and the health visitor's role is to help them enjoy it as much as possible. If the mother is feeling down it will be difficult for her to find pleasure in her baby.

The baby will also be part of the assessment. Mothers who are depressed often have babies who are difficult to soothe, feed and/or settle and they may avoid eye contact. Some babies are more difficult than others, but these features of the relationship may represent the baby's response to a depressed mother.

Assessment of suicide risk

Suicidal thoughts are extremely common and may occur at any point in a depressive illness. When asked, many people will admit to such thoughts but add, spontaneously, that they would not do it. It is important that questions are asked sensitively in language appropriate to the patient since there could be a risk of causing distress to a patient who has never had thoughts of suicide. More often, any discomfort in asking such questions is that of the professional, not the patient. Patients who are suicidal may experience considerable relief at being given 'permission' to express their feelings.

Notwithstanding the difficulties, the risk of suicide should be assessed by a nurse or doctor for every patient with depression, both as part of the initial assessment and on a regular basis during treatment. Suicidal ideas and thoughts volunteered spontaneously should never be ignored. It is not true that people who talk about suicide do not do it. They do.

In assessing risk, the following series of questions may be useful.

- Ideas (Do you feel that life is not worth living any more? Have you thought about harming yourself?)
- Intentions (Do you think you might act on these ideas?)
- Plans (Have you made any plans?)
- Previous attempts (Have you tried before?)

The person who has definite intentions to end his/her life and has made a plan is at high risk, especially if he/she has tried and failed previously. This should be regarded as a medical emergency and urgent referral to specialist care is required. Suicidal thoughts or ideas in the absence of intentions and/or plans represent a relatively low risk, but these patients still require monitoring and supporting, especially in the early weeks of treatment.

It is probably not advisable for primary care nurses to make a formal assessment for suicide risk except in the context of a practice policy or protocol. One of the ways of reducing professional stress about suicide is to be clear about the procedure to be followed in the worst case scenario. A useful exercise for a whole primary care team might be to think about the worst thing that could happen with a suicidal patient, and then to discuss what each member of the team should do in such a circumstance. It will probably never happen – but it helps to know what to do if it does.

Protocols for assessment of suicide risk are a requirement for all primary care teams under the National Service Framework for Mental Health. They need to include not only what should happen within a practice, but also referral criteria for specialist care including 24-hour crisis arrangements. Locums need to be aware of the system, as do local out-of-hours cooperatives.

It is not possible to identify those who are likely to kill themselves with any degree of accuracy but some groups are known to be particularly at risk. These include:

- older men who are unmarried, separated or widowed
- people with serious physical illness
- people with concurrent alcohol or substance misuse
- where there is a family history of suicide
- where the patient has tried before.

There has been a great deal of concern about the increase in the suicide rate amongst young men. The reasons for the increase are not clear and a variety of explanations have been proposed. Unemployment is almost certainly a factor. AIDS has also been cited as a possible cause. Men, at least in the west, have been disproportionately affected by AIDS and HIV and, as with any life-threatening illness, there is an increased risk of concurrent depression. Others have suggested that a contributory factor may be an increase in the number of boys being brought up by their mothers in single-parent households, depriving them of appropriate male role models. Alcohol and drug misuse, which are more common in males than females, may also have a part to play. The picture is complex.

Young men are difficult for primary care professionals to reach, since they consult their GP much less than young women. Nevertheless, when opportunities do arise, it is important to remember that men do become depressed and to ask appropriate questions. Opportunistic screening may be useful, especially for those known to be in high-risk groups.

People who repeatedly harm themselves, for example by overdoses or cutting, pose particular problems in primary care settings. They can be difficult to help. This phenomenon may be known as deliberate self-harm or parasuicide. Such acts may be seen as suicide attempts, though the person may not have an intention to die. Nevertheless, it is important to be aware that about 1% of people who attempt suicide and fail, go on to succeed within a year.[13] Concurrent abuse of alcohol or drugs will increase the risk.

Primary care teams may find it useful to develop a protocol for people who self-harm, jointly with their community mental health team so that the care may be shared. It can also be helpful to have the Samaritans National Helpline number displayed in the waiting area of the surgery. Local branches should be able to supply posters and cards.

Assessment tools

There are a number of well-researched and validated questionnaires which could be used with people who may be depressed. They can be used as an aid to diagnosis, to assess severity and to monitor progress and they can also be useful in clinical audit. They may be used as screening tools, particularly for people who are known to be at risk. For the nurse they may be helpful in making credible referrals to the GP. Using a scale may be seen as similar to using a peak flow meter in asthma.

For the patient, questionnaires may help to normalise the condition. If someone has taken the trouble to design a questionnaire, then other people must have suffered from this problem. Most scales used in primary care are short (12–15 questions) and are designed to be completed by the patient with minimal staff involvement.

The most commonly used scales are:

- Goldberg General Health Questionnaire (GHQ – 12 question version) – known as a global measure of distress. It does not diagnose depression. There are longer versions which have more specific questions.
- Hospital Anxiety and Depression Scale (HADS) – this scale has been validated for primary care use. It provides scores for both depression and anxiety.
- Geriatric Depression Scale (GDS) – many nurses find this scale useful as part of the over-75 health check.

- Edinburgh Postnatal Depression Scale (EPDS) – normally used by health visitors, it does not diagnose depression but assesses the frequency of symptoms.
- Beck Depression Inventory (BDI) – occasionally used in primary care but more often by specialists.

For details of availability, *see* Appendix.

Scales such as these should be used only for the appropriate population group and in the context of a whole primary care team approach. No scale replaces the need for a full clinical assessment. It is important that there are agreed routes of referral for those people whose score may indicate a need for something more than primary care treatment. Training in the use of scales is essential to avoid misuse, abuse and misinterpretation.

Treatment of depression

Treatment begins with recognition and acknowledgement. It is important to listen to, and to understand, the patient's beliefs about their symptoms, to accept that physical symptoms are real and a part of the illness and to offer acceptable explanations about symptoms which reflect the patient's experiences. For example, it can be helpful to relate the illness to recent life events or chronic problems.

As in any area of healthcare, it is essential to distinguish erroneous health beliefs which may be damaging, from those that are culturally different. This can present huge problems for primary care professionals especially in localities where there are large numbers of patients/clients from widely differing ethnic backgrounds. Nevertheless, some understanding of the patient's view of his/her problem and expectations of treatment must be sought if care is to be acceptable and effective. With non-English speaking patients, properly trained health interpreters should be used wherever possible (*see* Chapter 8).

Treatments fall into three main categories: drugs, talking treatments and self-help. Most people will benefit from a combination of approaches rather than either one or the other. Medication, appropriately prescribed, will improve symptoms but it will not treat social and emotional difficulties. There are potential roles for nurses in all aspects of treatment and care.

Medication

Antidepressant drugs work by increasing the levels of neurotransmitters in the brain, mainly serotonin, which are involved in the regulation of mood and emotions. Some of the newest antidepressants also increase levels of noradrenaline. All antidepressants are equally effective and most take between two and three weeks before they begin to have an effect on mood. All antidepressants need to be continued for at least four to six months after the patient begins to feel better to avoid the danger of relapse. The main differences between the drugs lie in their side effect profiles, hence their acceptability and their toxicity.

There are two main groups in common use in primary care. The older tricyclic antidepressants (TCAs) are well known and cheap, but their side effects tend to be unpleasant and may be intolerable, particularly at therapeutic dose. Some TCAs have cardiotoxic effects which may make them unsuitable for older patients and those with cardiovascular disease. They may also be sedating, and whilst this may be helpful for some people where sleep is a problem, others may find the drowsiness unacceptable. The sedative effect may also contribute to a risk of falls in older people. This group of drugs is highly toxic in overdose. A major problem with the TCAs is that the dose needs to be titrated upwards to reach the therapeutic level. Many patients do not reach this dosage, which calls into question the effectiveness of the prescription.

The newer selective serotonin re-uptake inhibitors (SSRIs) do have side effects, some of them unpleasant, but they appear to be better tolerated. They are less toxic in overdose than the TCAs and non-sedating. However, they may increase anxiety levels, at least in the first few days of treatment, and withdrawal (discontinuation) effects may be a problem. Generally, they are more expensive than the TCAs. As more of these drugs become available as generic preparations, cost comparisons between the groups will be less important.

Table 1.1 summarises the drugs in common use in primary care, together with their therapeutic dose. *Hypericum* (St John's Wort) is also included since it is known to be effective in mild to moderate depression. It is widely available in health food shops and is now being prescribed by some GPs. It should not be combined with any other antidepressants. As with any drug, herbal or otherwise, it does have side effects. It has some features in common with SSRIs and some with monoamine oxidase inhibitors (MAOIs). There are suggestions that some people may experience reactions with some foods, particularly red wine and cheese.

Table 1.1 Common antidepressants

Drug class	Examples with usual therapeutic dose range
Tricyclic antidepressants (TCAs)	Amitriptyline 125–150 mg at night Dothiepin 75–150 mg at night
Newer type TCAs	Lofepramine 140–210 mg daily
Selective serotonin re-uptake inhibitors (SSRIs)	Citalopram 20 mg daily Fluoxetine 20 mg daily Paroxetine 20–50 mg daily Sertraline 50–150 mg daily
Serotonin and noradrenaline re-uptake inhibitor (SNRI)	Venlafaxine 75–150 mg daily
Serotonin re-uptake inhibitor and serotonin receptor blocker	Nefazodone 100–200 mg twice daily
Noradrenergic and specific serotonergic antidepressant (NaSSA)	Mirtazepine 15–45 mg daily
Noradrenaline re-uptake inhibitor	Reboxetine 4 mg twice daily
Lithium	Lithium 400–1000 mg daily
Monoamine oxidase inhibitors (MAOIs)	Phenelzine 15 mg three times daily
Reversible inhibitor of monoamine oxidase (RIMA)	Moclobemide 150–600 mg daily
St John's Wort (*Hypericum perforatum*)	300–1000 mg extract daily

Adapted from Northamptonshire Health Authority 1998.[14]

Recently there have been warnings that it should not be taken with some cardiovascular medications.

There are differences both between the groups and between individual drugs within the groups and the decision on which drug to prescribe needs to take the patient's life style into account. The main differences are summarised in Table 1.2.

Patients require information about their medication. Verbal information at the time of the consultation is rarely adequate since most people will remember very little of what is said. Back up leaflets, audiotapes or even videos may be helpful and should be available. Patients prescribed antidepressants also require regular follow up and monitoring (*see* WHO Guide), including re-assessment of suicide risk. There may be some increase in suicide risk around the third or fourth week of treatment when

Table 1.2 Characteristics of antidepressants

Drug class	Advantages	Disadvantages
TCAs	Cheap Long experience in use Side effects known Sedative effects may be helpful for some patients	Toxic in overdose. Anticholinergic side effects may be intolerable, e.g. dry mouth, blurred vision, constipation, urinary retention May be cardiotoxic Need to build up slowly to therapeutic dose
Lofepramine	Safer in overdose Less cardiotoxic and less sedating than older drugs Cheaper than newer drugs	Anticholinergic side effects as above, but may be less severe
SSRIs	May be better tolerated than older drugs Less sedating and less toxic in overdose than older drugs	Short-term increase in anxiety symptoms may be unacceptable Gastrointestinal side effects, dizziness, headaches More expensive than TCAs but some now available as generic preparations
Other newer drugs	As effective as other drugs, venlafaxine may have better side effect profile Sexual dysfunction appears to be uncommon with nefazodone	Still need more comparative data and data on long-term use
Lithium	Mood stabiliser mainly used in bipolar disorder May be useful in recurrent depression	Highly toxic. Regular blood checks and checks of kidney and thyroid function are required
Monoamine oxidase inhibitors (MAOIs)	Useful when other antidepressants have failed	Toxic effects with tyramine-containing foods which must be avoided, e.g. cheese, pickled herring, broad bean pods, meat and yeast extracts Normally used by specialists Should not be given with other antidepressants

Cont.

Moclobemide	Claimed to have less toxic effects with tyramine-containing foods	Patients should still be advised to avoid large amounts of cheese etc Should not be given with other antidepressants
St John's Wort	Evidence that this extract is effective in mild to moderate depression	More research needed especially into toxicity Recent reports of interactions with cardiovascular drugs Some side effects common to both SSRIs and MAOIs

Adapted from Northamptonshire Health Authority 1998.[14]

motivation begins to improve, but mood may not have lifted greatly. Follow-up and monitoring does not have to be done by a doctor. Some nurses have developed collaborative schemes with GP colleagues.[15] Many professionals believe that antidepressants should not be prescribed on repeat prescriptions.

Antidepressants are not addictive, but patients may experience discontinuation effects if the drug is stopped suddenly. For this reason the WHO Guidelines recommend that all antidepressant drugs should be withdrawn slowly over a period of at least four weeks. Patients need to be monitored for these effects, and for signs of relapse.

Most people with severe depression, including severe postnatal depression, will require treatment with antidepressants. Progestogens are not effective in the treatment of postnatal depression. A recent review suggests that their use may be associated with increased depressive symptoms at six weeks post-partum.[16] Evidence to date suggests no major problems with the use of SSRI antidepressants in breast-feeding mothers,[17] but advice may be required from specialists.

Nurses may play an important role in helping patients understand the way the medication works, advising on coping with side effects in the early weeks of treatment and in reinforcing the need to take the drugs for an adequate length of time. There are a number of factors which are known to predict non-adherence to treatment:

- patient health beliefs; attitude to medication; previous experience of medication
- attitudes of family and friends
- negative attitudes associated with depressive illness

- treatment regime, e.g. frequency of dose and ease of following the regime
- behaviour and attitudes of professionals advising on treatment
- the context in which treatment is delivered.

Adapted from Peveler 1999.[18]

A brief counselling-type intervention used by practice nurses which was designed to modify these factors, was shown to improve treatment adherence and patient outcome in patients taking therapeutic doses of antidepressants.[19]

Talking treatments

There are several psychological techniques which have been shown to be effective in the treatment of depression, mainly cognitive behavioural therapy (CBT) and problem solving. In postnatal depression, techniques derived from Rogerian counselling, especially active reflective listening, have been shown to work.[20] The beneficial effects of this are also likely to be apparent in other patients with depression. For nurses, it may be difficult to learn to put aside the need to give advice or to do something to relieve the patient's pain. Simply being there, listening and acknowledging the distress is more important.

Tools and methods derived from CBT, structured problem solving, solution focused therapy and related disciplines are widely used by primary care professionals, especially to help people with mild to moderate symptoms for whom antidepressants are less appropriate and for whom referral to secondary care services is not an option. This group forms an important part of the primary care clientele, but their response to the various talking treatments available has been much less studied than that of people with major depression. Unless primary care nurses and others learn to use some of the available techniques, there is a serious danger that many distressed people will receive no help at all.[21] The evidence suggests that many will recover eventually anyway, but others will go on to develop chronic conditions and become high users of practice time. Chapter 3 gives a practical view of how some of these techniques may be adapted and used by nurses in primary care settings.

It has been suggested that a crucial part of any intervention for depression should be helping people access social support, especially finding someone in whom they can confide. Although being willing to listen is a crucial part of any health professional's role, clearly it is impossible to be everybody's confidante. It is much more realistic to help people access the sources of support which exist in most communities, such as self-help organisations, befriending schemes and church or other religious groups.

Cognitive behavioural therapy

The style of thinking of people with depression has been described in terms of a 'cognitive triad':

- negative perception of self – 'I'm useless'
- negative interpretation of experiences – 'Nothing good ever happens to me'
- negative view of the future – 'It'll never get any better'.

These negative thoughts arise because of errors in processing perceptions and interpretations of experiences, leading to distortion. Depressed people pay more attention to those events and experiences that reinforce their feelings of defeat and inadequacy.

Cognitive therapy attempts to help people recognise and question these negative thoughts, replacing them with more realistic and positive alternatives. Patients will also learn to challenge unhelpful attitudes which have arisen from past experience.

A full course of CBT provided by a clinical psychologist or trained therapist may take between 15 and 30 hours, but there is a shortage of therapists and waiting lists tend to be very lengthy. However, many of the techniques can be learned by primary care professionals and may be useful in brief therapy more suited to the primary care setting. CBT techniques are becoming available through interactive computer-based programs. These have been shown to be acceptable to patients, but systems may be expensive and are not widely accessible as yet.

Structured problem solving

This is a useful technique which is used with success by some practice nurses. Health visitors often use a version of it with their clients.

Structured problem solving has been shown to be effective in the treatment of people with major depression, especially once they have started to respond to medication, but it is also helpful for use with less depressed patients who have a number of problems which are contributing to a level of distress.

Counselling

Counselling may be especially useful for patients who have specific problems such as interpersonal difficulties, family problems and bereavement. Patients should be referred to an appropriately trained counsellor or agency skilled in their particular problem. The Association of Counsellors and Psychotherapists in Primary Care (*see* Appendix) maintains a register of counsellors who meet appropriate criteria in terms of training and supervision. Many practices have their own counsellors on site, most of whom, nowadays, will have adequate training. It will be necessary for the primary care team to discuss with the counsellor his/her techniques or special areas of expertise. Lack of communication and understanding will lead to inappropriate referrals and the best use will not be made of what may be a scarce resource.

Counselling involves a number of one-to-one sessions with a trained counsellor. The number may vary from one to about 12, with an average of six. Sessions normally last about 50 minutes. In the first session, the counsellor will assess the suitability of the client for counselling and establish a therapeutic alliance, seeking to understand the problems the client brings and exploring their life history to understand the context. The counsellor will check any medication the client is taking, and make a risk assessment.

The sessions will enable a greater understanding of the problem and will look at areas of acceptance and areas of change. The counselling aims to equip the client to take a more constructive approach to difficult issues in their life. Counselling can improve physical symptoms such as inability to sleep, anxiety, headaches and low mood.

Early research into the effectiveness of counselling in primary care was inconclusive, but most reviews acknowledged that there were severe limitations in many of the studies for a variety of reasons which included small sample sizes, inadequate outcome measures and difficulties in describing the interventions which were being tested. Mellor-Clark believes that the situation is improving due to better methods of measurement, and that the evidence of effectiveness is growing.[22]

For people with multiple practical difficulties such as debt, unemployment or housing problems, referral to a social worker, debt advice agency or Citizen's Advice Bureau may be appropriate.

Patient information and education

One of the commonest causes of treatment failure (and inappropriate referrals to secondary care) is said to be poor treatment adherence due to inadequate information, education and support. This situation can be improved. The use of written back up or other information has already been mentioned in connection with medication but it is also crucial for people with less severe illnesses who are not taking medication. Some sources of good quality information about depression are listed in the Appendix. Nurses are well used to providing information to patients and could take on the role of ensuring that patients with depression understand their illness, their treatment and how to get the best from it.

Self-help

Good treatment for depression includes attention to physical health. People may need to be encouraged to eat healthily, avoid alcohol, which is a depressant, and, as they begin to recover, to gradually increase the amount of exercise they take. It is useful to help people set achievable goals for each day or each week. Alternative therapies such as aromatherapy, reflexology or relaxation may be useful because they increase a feeling of well being, though they will not treat the depressive symptoms. Self-help groups, whilst they will not suit everyone, can be a very much valued source of support and information for many people. Depression Alliance, and other voluntary agencies, run self-help groups nationwide.

Carer support

Depression affects not just the sufferer, but also their family and friends. Immediate carers particularly may need information and support. In some instances it may be helpful to see close members of the family in the practice to ensure that they also understand the illness. Again, Depression Alliance may be helpful, and there are books written especially for carers.

Effective care and treatment for people with depressive illness is rewarding for primary care teams because most people will recover. However, it may also be stressful to professionals, particularly if they feel unsupported by colleagues. There is a danger that if only one person within a team has an interest in depression, that person will become overloaded and burnt out. Further chapters in this book will look at ways of developing a team approach to this problem. It should be possible to create within most practice premises an atmosphere which promotes mental health and well being for staff as well as patients.

References

1   Paykel ES and Priest RG (1992) Recognition and management of depression in general practice: consensus statement. *BMJ*. **305**: 1198–202.

2   Ballard CG, Stanley AK and Brockington IF (1995) Post Traumatic Stress Disorder (PTSD) after childbirth. *Br J Psychiatry*. **68**(5): 185–7.

3   Gilbert P (1992) *Depression. The evolution of powerlessness* (Chapter 2). Lawrence Erlbaum Associates, Hove.

4   Wilkinson G, Moore B and Moore P (1999) *Treating People with Depression: a practical guide for primary care*. Radcliffe Medical Press, Oxford.

5   France R and Robson M (1997) *Cognitive Behavioural Therapy in Primary Care* (Chapter 5). Jessica Kingsley Publishers, London.

6   Jenkins R (1992) Depression and anxiety: an overview of preventive strategies. In: R Jenkins, J Newton and R Youngs (eds) *The Prevention of Depression and Anxiety: the role of the primary care team*. HMSO, London.

7   Parkes CM (1986) *Bereavement: studies of grief in adult life*. Penguin Books, London.

8   Sharp D (1996) The prevention of postnatal depression. In: T Kendrick, A Tylee and P Freeling (eds) *The Prevention of Mental Illness in Primary Care*. Cambridge University Press, Cambridge.

9   Sheppard M (1997) Depression in female health visitor consulters: social and demographic factors. *J Adv Nurs*. **26**: 921–9.

10 Tylee A (1996) The secondary prevention of depression. In: T Kendrick, A Tylee and P Freeling (eds) *The Prevention of Mental Illness in Primary Care*. Cambridge University Press, Cambridge.

11 Hook A (1994) A framework for consultation. *Practice Nursing.* **5**(17): 37–8.

12 Murray L and Cooper PJ (eds) (1997) *Postpartum Depression and Child Development.* Guilford Press, New York.

13 Roberts D (1996) Suicide prevention by general nurses. *Nursing Standard.* **10**(7): 30–3.

14 Northamptonshire GRiPP (Getting Research into Practice and Purchasing) Project (1998) *Guidelines for the Recognition and Management of Depression in Primary Care.* Northamptonshire Health Authority.

15 Gardner S (1999) Practice nurses in mental health: a changing role? *J Primary Care Mental Health.* **2**: 11–12.

16 Lawrie TA, Herxheimer A and Dalton K (1999) Oestrogens and progestogens for preventing and treating postnatal depression. Cochrane Review. In: *The Cochrane Library.* Update Software, Oxford.

17 Misri S, Burgmann A and Kostaras D (2000) Are SSRIs safe for pregnant and breast feeding women? *Can Fam Physician.* **46**: 626–8, 631–3.

18 Peveler R (1999) Encouraging concordance with treatment for depression and schizophrenia. *Community Ment Health.* **2**(3): 5–7.

19 Peveler R, George C, Kinmoth A-L *et al.* (1999) Effect of antidepressant drug counselling and information leaflets on adherence to drug treatment in primary care: randomised controlled trial. *BMJ.* **319**: 612–15.

20 Holden JM, Sagovsky R and Cox JL (1987) Counselling in a general practice setting: controlled study of health visitor intervention in treatment of postnatal depression. *BMJ.* **298**: 223–6.

21 Clinical Standards Advisory Group (1999) *Services for Patients with Depression.* Department of Health, London.

22 Mellor-Clark J (2000) *Counselling in Primary Care in the Context of the NHS Quality Agenda. The facts.* British Association for Counselling and Psychotherapy, Rugby.

Further reading

Bhugra D and Bahl V (1999) *Ethnicity: an agenda for mental health.* Gaskell, London.

Cooper PJ and Murray L (1998) Postnatal depression (fortnightly review). *BMJ.* **316**: 1884–7.

Gilbert P (1992) *Depression. The evolution of powerlessness.* Lawrence Erlbaum Associates, Hove.

Murray J (1995) *Prevention of Anxiety and Depression in Vulnerable Groups.* Gaskell, London.

Wilkinson G, Moore B and Moore P (1999) *Treating People with Depression: a practical guide for primary care.* Radcliffe Medical Press, Oxford.

CHAPTER TWO

Anxiety, stress and related conditions

Martin Davies and Elizabeth Armstrong

Like depression, anxiety is a normal experience. Everyone feels anxious from time to time, particularly in stressful situations such as an examination, a difficult task at work or a personal or family crisis. This anxiety may lead to symptoms like headache or gastric upsets, dry mouth, sweating, palpitations or shallow, rapid breathing. It may be hard to relax or get to sleep. People may become irritable and snap at colleagues or family members with little obvious cause. People commonly understand that an emotional outburst of anger or inappropriate laughter may be due to 'stress'.

The term 'stress' is vague and can be difficult to define. Everyone interprets it differently. It could be seen as the individual's perception of the pressure upon them, or the 'three way relationship between demands on a person, that person's feelings about those demands, and their ability to cope with those demands'.[1] Normal stress, that is stress that is proportionate to the situation, is a biologically protective experience. It draws attention to oncoming danger and, unless overwhelming, promotes a state of physical and psychological readiness.[2]

It is clear, therefore, that not all stress is harmful. Some stress seems to be necessary for optimal functioning. It can provide motivation and lead to worthwhile change.[3] Short-term stress generally improves performance, providing a heightened sense of alertness and what some people call a 'buzz'. However, if the stress levels are maintained, or increased over time, this can lead to 'burnout' at best, but for some people it can also lead to depression. The range of experiences can be viewed as a continuum:

Normal stress → anxiety/depression

Arousal – unease – distress – fear/terror

The extent to which stress results from various demands is also linked to how well a person is doing at any particular time in their life. Something which might be stressful at a time of turmoil could be seen as an enjoyable challenge in happier times.[4]

It is also important to realise that stress is the common component of all mental illnesses – managing most mental illness depends largely on managing the individual's stress and tension. Although the person suffering from schizophrenia, manic depression, anorexia or depression may require medication, it is the importance of teaching the individual to manage his/her own levels of emotional arousal that provides the basis for good self-management and relapse prevention.

It has been suggested that up to a quarter of patients attending their GP may have anxiety symptoms, but research into anxiety at primary care level is sparse. Recent epidemiological studies show that the most common experience appears to be a mixed anxiety/depression syndrome.[5] In older people particularly, anxiety or agitation may be a prominent feature of a depressive illness. People with anxiety should always be assessed for depression. Where depression is present, this should be treated as the primary illness.[6] Treating anxiety first may lead to inappropriate use of benzodiazepines such as diazepam, which are highly addictive. Antidepressants are not addictive, and some are anxiolytic – that is, they treat anxiety as well as depression.

Anxiety is common in children, and, as with depression, the way the disorder presents is likely to vary according to the stage of development of the child. Anxious children will often complain of physical symptoms such as abdominal pain. They may present with enuresis – especially a child who has previously been dry – or there may be exacerbations of health problems such as asthma or eczema. Behavioural problems may also be a feature.

The diagnosis of anxiety

In the WHO Guide, anxiety is classified under a number of different headings.

- Generalised anxiety is excessive worry about life circumstances and social difficulties. It may have been present for several months by the time the patient arrives at their GP surgery. The diagnostic features are:

     – *physical arousal* including dizziness, sweating, fast or pounding heart, dry mouth, stomach pains, chest pains

     – *mental tension* including worry, feeling tense or nervous, poor concentration, fear that something dangerous is about to happen and that the patient will not be able to cope with it

     – *physical tension* including restlessness, headaches, tremors, inability to relax.

    These symptoms may be triggered by a stressful event, but may persist where there are chronic social difficulties.

- Panic attacks are sudden, unexplained attacks of anxiety symptoms which develop rapidly and often last only a few minutes. They can be extremely frightening and include physical sensations such as palpitations, chest pain, choking feelings, churning stomach, dizziness and feelings of unreality. Patients often fear that they will lose control or go mad and may also fear a heart attack or other personal disaster.

    One panic attack may lead to fear of another or to avoidance of places where a previous attack happened.

- Phobias are irrational or unreasonably strong fears of people, places, things or events. Many people have minor phobias, particularly of animals or insects, but whilst they will take steps to avoid the object of the fear, other aspects of social functioning are unaffected. Phobias only come to the attention of the doctor when they are severe enough to disrupt the person's life.

    Agoraphobia is the best known of the severe phobias. It involves fear of crowded places such as supermarkets as well as open spaces. Fear of leaving home may also be a feature. Social phobias such as fear of answering the telephone or of eating in public places may be severely distressing to a person whose job depends on meeting people. These fears, usually of doing something embarrassing or humiliating in public, often arise in the teenage years. Depression is commonly associated with such conditions.

- Obsessive-compulsive disorder involves recurrent, intrusive thoughts which lead to repetitive behaviour. The individual is aware that the obsessive thoughts are absurd and are leading to compulsive behaviour such as excessive cleaning or hand washing. Attempts to resist the urges cause extreme tension and anxiety which is only relieved by giving in to the urge. The behaviour then becomes a ritual which may severely disrupt the individual's life.

Obsessive-compulsive disorder (OCD) seems to be more common than was once believed, and it is now considered to be linked to a disturbance in brain function.[6]

- Post-traumatic stress disorder (PTSD) is the name now given to a psychological reaction to an extremely distressing or catastrophic event, whose nature is severe enough to cause marked distress to anyone. It is not a new condition but has been known for many years under various names, for example, shell shock or combat neurosis. It is characterised by repeated flashbacks and/or nightmares about the trauma, emotional numbness and detachment from other people and avoidance of situations which remind the person about the trauma. There may also be autonomic hyperarousal with enhanced startle reaction, hypervigilance and insomnia.

The onset of PTSD is usually delayed for days or months following the traumatic event. Some have suggested that the delay might even last many years in some instances. For example, it seems that some elderly men and women are only now acknowledging symptoms of PTSD related to extreme war-time experiences going back to the Second World War and the Korean war of the 1950s.

Only a proportion of those experiencing an extreme trauma will develop PTSD, suggesting that there may also be vulnerability factors at work. It seems to be important to distinguish true PTSD from the symptoms of an adjustment disorder or reaction which may follow any psychological trauma or severe life event.

There are suggestions that PTSD following childbirth may be more common than usually supposed. Robinson suggests that the Edinburgh Postnatal Depression Scale does not distinguish between postnatal depression and PTSD, and may contribute to under-diagnosis.[7]

Causes of anxiety

Anxiety may be a perfectly normal response to particular stressful situations. It only becomes an illness when it is more severe than the situation would appear to warrant, or occurs when there is no obvious threat. In such a case, there is usually a combination of physical and psychological symptoms which affect all systems of the body. It is important to recognise and acknowledge that all the symptoms are real. They are not imaginary. They may occur as separate attacks or as a persistent state.

In some instances, anxiety symptoms may be a learned response to situations which would not normally seem threatening. Cognitive theory suggests that anxiety disorders may persist because of the way some people think about their symptoms, for example, fear about symptoms may lead to more anxiety, with the subsequent development of a vicious circle.

A number of physical illnesses may cause anxiety symptoms. In some cases this may be because of understandable worries about the illness, but in other instances anxiety symptoms may be an integral part of the condition. Examples include thyrotoxicosis and some other endocrine diseases, some cardiovascular, respiratory or neurological disorders. Treatment of the underlying condition may relieve the anxiety.

Anxiety may be related to medication, prescribed or otherwise. Prescribed drugs which may cause anxiety include corticosteroids, bronchodilators, ephedrine, amphetamines and thyroxine. It has been suggested that excessive caffeine intake is an important and frequently overlooked cause of symptoms of anxiety at primary care level. Anxiety symptoms are also a feature of withdrawal from benzodiazepines and this may lead to an erroneous belief that the original illness has recurred. Patients withdrawing from these drugs need information and support. Alcohol and cigarettes may be used as inappropriate ways of coping with anxiety symptoms, but instead of helping they are likely to make symptoms worse.

Causes may be obvious or difficult to establish. The priority is to take the patient's symptoms seriously regardless of the cause. Identifying the cause can be helpful, particularly in seeing how the present symptoms have arisen and how they may be maintained.[6,8] In summary, the following are worth considering:

- **Life events**   Life trauma (bereavement, other loss); life changes and transitions; high expectations, demands and responsibility; relationship conflicts, etc.
- **Learned behaviours**   Insecure children; anxious parents; inconsistent parenting; established inadequate or inappropriate coping methods.
- **Hereditary factors**   Personality traits and family history.
- **Support**   Poor support, lack of confiding relationships.
- **Health**   Chronic emotional and physical health problems.

Assessment

Appropriate treatment depends on careful assessment. Because of the similarity and overlap of symptoms, it is easy to believe that the person may be suffering from anxiety when, in fact, it may be depression.[9] The opposite is also true. It is useful to run through the following checklist:

- **Severity:** How bad is it? (You may wish to use a 0–10 scale).
- **Duration:** How long have you felt like this?
- **Past history:** Have you ever felt like this before? What was happening at that time in your life?
- **Family history:** Has anyone else in the family had similar difficulties?
- **Support:** Have you talked to someone, a friend or member of your family about how you have been feeling? Are you still seeing your friends as much as you have in the past? Do you have a good friend to talk to?
- **Self-esteem:** Do you feel as confident as you have always been?
- **Avoidance:** Are there any places, events, people or situations that you have found yourself avoiding because of the feelings that you have been experiencing?
- **Biological symptoms:** Questions about sleep, appetite, concentration, physical aches or pains, headaches, feelings of fear or apprehension.
- **Alcohol/drugs:** Are you drinking any more that you normally do? How much and what? Are you taking any medications, herbal remedies or other 'leisure' drugs? How much and what? How much coffee/tea do you drink?

Assessment tools

A helpful assessment tool to clarify the severity and highlight the main problem is the HAD scale (*see* Chapter 1). This is a 14-item questionnaire that assesses both anxiety and depression. It takes about 5 minutes for the patient to complete and the advantages can be:

- it helps the patient acknowledge the problem
- it is easy and understandable
- it is not as threatening as asking what may seem to be embarrassing or awkward questions
- it is validated and evidence based

Box 2.1   CAGE Questionnaire

1   Have you ever felt that you should **CUT** down on your drinking?
2   Have people **ANNOYED** you by criticising your drinking?
3   Have you ever felt bad or **GUILTY** about your drinking?
4   Have you ever had a drink first thing in the morning to steady your nerves or get rid of a hangover? (**EYE-OPENER**)

- it clarifies the initial diagnosis
- it provides a monitoring device (repeat it at intervals as appropriate)
- it can consolidate a referral to the GP or other member of the team
- it can save time.

The HADS can easily be incorporated into the consultation. It is important to remember that if the problem appears to be depression, a full assessment of depression needs to be made. This assessment must include an assessment of level of risk, especially suicide risk. The HADS can help provide a standardised approach to the assessment of anxiety and depression.

The CAGE questionnaire (Box 2.1) may be useful to assess alcohol intake. This questionnaire may be familiar to nurses from the assessment of drinking habits for physical health reasons. It is important to remember that excessive use of alcohol has important adverse effects on psychological as well as physical health and may severely disrupt relationships and social functioning.[10]

A thorough assessment will help the nurse to decide whether GP or other referral is necessary. Patients with severe anxiety symptoms, or severe depression with anxiety, should always be referred. People with milder symptoms will probably not need referral, but may be helped by a straightforward acknowledgement of the problem, some appropriate explanation and the use of some of the techniques which will be described in the following chapter.

Treatment of anxiety

As with depression, treatment begins with recognition and acknowledgement. Anxious patients often fear that they have a serious physical illness even where no evidence of this can be found. Patients' beliefs about their symptoms must be listened to, and the reality of the symptoms accepted. Explanations about the causes of anxiety symptoms will be important. Cultural aspects are as important here as in depression. There are considerable problems with research into mental illness in ethnic minority groups. Research has often been undertaken from a western standpoint, which, many believe, makes it difficult to interpret.[11] Any conclusions may, at best, be misleading if not completely erroneous.

From a practical nursing standpoint, it would seem to be important to adopt a questioning and listening attitude, asking the patient to help the nurse understand what is happening to them, and what this means to the patient and their family.

Medication is rarely a first line treatment for anxiety symptoms. Enabling the patient to learn skills to deal with the symptoms and triggers is far more important. Because of the dangers of dependency, benzodiazepines are advised only for the short-term treatment (2–4 weeks) of severe, disabling anxiety symptoms. Likewise these drugs should only be used for insomnia when it is causing the patient severe distress.

Many antidepressants are effective in treating anxiety, including the SSRIs which may be used for long-term treatment. However, the SSRIs may be associated with a temporary increase in anxiety symptoms early in treatment. Patients need to be warned what to expect and be encouraged to persevere. The SNRI, venlafaxine, is now licensed for use in generalised anxiety. Drug treatment alone is unlikely to be sufficient. For best results it is likely that it will need to be combined with some form of psychological treatment.

People with severe anxiety and disabling phobias will most likely require specialist psychological therapy which may be available from suitably trained community psychiatric nurses, clinical nurse therapists or clinical psychology departments. Some form of behavioural therapy is the most usual approach. These therapies are based on learning theory and may include exposing the patient to a feared situation in a controlled manner. Exposure may be rapid ('exposure in vivo', previously known as 'flooding') or gradual ('graded exposure' or 'desensitisation').[12]

Exposure in vivo involves the therapist accompanying the patient into the feared situation and remaining there until the patient's symptoms subside. With practice, the patient learns to control the anxiety even in the absence of the therapist. This method normally requires a trained and experienced professional counsellor, psychologist or nurse therapist.

Graded exposure involves breaking down the task into small, manageable steps. These work on a hierarchical principle, where a series of goals contribute towards finally confronting the situation which is most feared. A reward system may be built in so that achievement of each goal adds to the improvement of self-esteem. Though this method is suitable for use at home, it requires great commitment by patient, relatives and therapist. Well-structured anxiety management approaches need to address the following issues:

- somatic symptoms
- cognitive symptoms
- avoidance
- low self-confidence.

Nurses in primary care, especially practice nurses, need to be aware of any patient undergoing this form of treatment in order to avoid undermining the therapist's work and the patient's progress. The unwary primary care professional may unwittingly accede to a request for medication by a patient who is finding the treatment hard going. A more constructive response would be support and encouragement to continue with the therapy.

In the past there has been a fashion for running anxiety management groups in primary care settings. To be effective, these require skilled and experienced leaders and are probably best run by specialists. In contrast, stress management groups may be within the skills of practice nurses or health visitors, though some extra training may be needed.

For people with milder symptoms of anxiety and stress, there are a variety of non-drug strategies which may be used by primary care nurses to help their patients. Many of these are of use in both anxiety and depression. They will be described in more detail in the next chapter.

Conclusion

Anxiety symptoms are common amongst people attending their GP surgery and amongst the patients and clients of primary care nurses. Referral for medication should only be necessary where the symptoms are very severe and disabling. For most people it will be more beneficial to learn appropriate coping strategies, many of which can be learned and taught by primary care nurses.

References

1   Richards C (1989) *The Health of Doctors*. King's Fund, London.

2   Trethowan W and Sims ACP (1983) *Psychiatry* (5e). Baillière Tindall, London.

3   Sutherland VJ and Cooper CL (1990) *Understanding Stress* (Chapter 5). Chapman & Hall, London.

4   Chambers R and Davies M (1999) *What Stress in Primary Care?* RCGP, London.

5   Meltzer H, Gill B and Petticrew M (1994) *The prevalence of psychiatric morbidity amongst adults aged 16–64, living in private households, in Great Britain*. OPCS, London.

6   Wilkinson G, Moore B and Moore P (2000) *Treating People with Anxiety and Stress: a practical guide for primary care*. Radcliffe Medical Press, Oxford.

7   Robinson J (1998) Suicide: a major cause of maternal deaths. *Br J Midwifery*. **6**(12): 767.

8   Marks IM (1969) *Fears and Phobias*. Heinemann Medical, London.

9   Casey PR (1993) *A Guide to Psychiatry in Primary Care* (Chapter 8). Wrightson Biomedical Publishing, Petersfield.

10   Williams H and Ghodse H (1996) The prevention of alcohol and drug misuse (Chapter 13). In: T Kendrick, A Tylee and P Freeling (eds) *The Prevention of Mental Illness in Primary Care*. Cambridge University Press, Cambridge.

11   Patel S (1996) Preventing mental illness amongst people of ethnic minorities (Chapter 6). In: T Kendrick, A Tylee and P Freeling (eds) *The Prevention of Mental Illness in Primary Care*. Cambridge University Press, Cambridge.

12   Armstrong E (1995) *Mental Health Issues in Primary Care: a practical guide* (Chapter 5). Macmillan, London.

Further reading

Marks I (1995) *Living with Fear*. McGraw-Hill, New York.

Priest R (1996) *Anxiety and Depression*. Century Vermillion, London.

Wilkinson G, Moore B and Moore P (2000) *Treating People with Anxiety and Stress: a practical guide for primary care*. Radcliffe Medical Press, Oxford.

CHAPTER THREE

Interventions for anxiety, stress and depression: skills for primary care nurses

Martin Davies

Introduction

It has long been recognised that the use of benzodiazepines (tranquillisers) can quickly produce addiction and longer-term problems for the sufferer. There is still an alarmingly high usage of sedation and sleeping tablets (which are usually benzodiazepines) which simply reduce some of the symptoms but should only be used for short periods unless specialist advice is sought.

There is no evidence that antidepressants are effective in mild depression. Moreover, many people are reluctant to take medication. Yet people with mild to moderate symptoms of anxiety and depression are a very important part of the primary care workload. These people cannot be dismissed as 'the worried well' and sent away. It may be more accurate to characterise them as 'worried sick'. They have come to the doctor or nurse for help. Nurses and other primary care professionals therefore need a 'toolkit' of ways of helping this large group of patients.

Helping people cope with stress-related problems, anxiety and depression involves:

- early recognition and acknowledgement
- understanding the symptoms
- assessment and review of life style; solving problems where possible
- modifying present coping strategies
- developing new coping strategies
- supporting, monitoring and reviewing.

Explaining the symptoms

There is little point in providing 'anxiety management', whatever form this may take, if no time is taken to explain to the patient how the symptoms arise and what they can and cannot do to the patient. The patient's own beliefs about this need to be explored and addressed. Once this explanation has been given in a manner that is understandable, then the approaches that are employed to help are logical. Many of the techniques applied in primary care, such as providing relaxation tapes and exercises, may be extremely wasteful, not only for the clinician but also for the patient, simply because no explanation took place at the beginning. A coping method is only going to be practised if there is a sound reason as to why it may be helpful.

Consider: if your car stopped running and you took it to a garage to be fixed, and the mechanic came out simply to say 'It's fixed' – would that be enough for you? Most people would certainly want to know why it stopped, how it occurred in the first place, and what they could do to prevent it happening again.

It is therefore not adequate to say 'You are suffering from stress and you need to practise the exercises on this audio tape once a day', then to give the patient a tape or a leaflet without further ado. Tapes and leaflets certainly have their place, but only after clear explanation and follow-up is provided by the nurse or doctor.

Dealing with panic: understanding the symptoms and reducing the fear

It is fundamental to understand how arousal can produce physical symptoms. Unless the sufferer understands what is happening, the fear may remain. The effects of adrenal stimulation should be explained in easy to understand language, and it should be clarified how simply thinking 'hot thoughts' can arouse the body physiologically. It is vital to explain that the short-term release of adrenaline cannot cause any harm – it might produce sensations that, if misinterpreted, may lead one to think that fainting is imminent, or that collapse is inevitable ... but feelings can tell lies! It might feel that your heart will burst or that your breathing will cause you to pass out – but they won't. Adrenaline surges tighten some muscles causing sensations (e.g. tightness, pain, discomfort), but that is all it is – a sensation that will cause no consequence. Adrenaline is a natural hormone and the body is well equipped to deal with it. Remember also that this hormone speeds up thinking processes, which, if one is thinking particularly fearful thoughts in the first place, can cause a 'rush' of fear and hence 'panic thinking'. It is important to try to 'catch' these thoughts early.

If no-one explains these symptoms and why they occur, it is understandable for a lay person to believe that they may be having a heart attack, or that collapse is imminent! Accident and emergency departments, as well as doctors' surgeries, are full of people who are simply misinterpreting their symptoms. The nurse's role therefore, is to help to clarify the symptoms so that no further misinterpretation takes place – this kind of explanation is intended for 'adoption' by the patient, equipping the sufferer with facts that can be turned into a kind of 'self-counselling' technique.

'Catching' it early!

This can be learned – watch out for 'troublesome' or 'fearful' thoughts. Practise saying 'STOP!' to these thoughts. For instance, when suddenly aware of a 'hot thought' you might say to yourself:

> 'STOP! Stop this thought RIGHT NOW! Don't let this thought through – don't wait for even a minute or so – stop it NOW! Come on . . . you know you need to catch this one . . . don't let it take hold. Try to move this thought onto something else . . . come on . . . try thinking about something else that is going on around you.'

Then follow this by:

> 'Good. Well done . . . you caught that one!'

Sometimes it might be easier for a person to instantly *do* something different as a distraction – an activity of some sort that is absorbing.

Distraction can be achieved in several ways:

- **Change behaviour:** Quickly do something different, walk away, carry out a physical exercise, talk to someone.

- **Mental imagery/visualisation:** Imagine a pleasant and relaxing scene (e.g. a previous holiday), listen to some music, talk yourself through an absorbing activity (e.g. a recipe or a mechanical technique).
- **Relaxation techniques:** Take one or two slow deep breaths ... relax your shoulders ... your arms ... your hands ... each of your fingers ... take a deep breath ... etc. It is also helpful to practise some deeper relaxation techniques (e.g. using an audio tape or CD instruction). Make sure these are practised when you feel relaxed so that when you are feeling tense, you can then bring your practised techniques into play.
- **Aromatherapy:** Try carrying around a couple of different essential oils that you favour (try *Geranium* or *Lavender* for instance). When you feel a bit tense, put a drop or two of an oil into a handkerchief or tissue and smell it. Practise this by using the same oils at home when you are relaxed, or try using them in your bath – create a pleasant association between the aroma and how they make you feel. Try different oils for different moods and feelings. In panic, we often do not use our sense of taste or smell – by suddenly overloading these 'unused' senses, our panic feelings can be quickly reduced. Use citrus flavours to overload the sense of taste.

Box 3.1   Ten steps to avoid panic

It can be helpful to carry a card around with you, with the following ten points on it. When we are tense it can be difficult to remember what we are supposed to be saying to ourselves. Use this as a 'prompt':

1   **Remember** that these feelings are nothing more than an exaggeration of the body's normal response to stress.
2   These feelings are **not harmful** or in the slightest way dangerous. They are uncomfortable or unpleasant, but they *cannot do anything to you.* They **will** pass.
3   Thinking frightening thoughts only adds to your sense of panic – adding more 'hot thoughts' just 'feeds' your sense of distress.
4   Try to describe slowly to yourself what is **really** happening to your body, not what you think is about to happen. Stick to the **facts**!

5   Allow some time to pass without fighting the feelings or running away. Try to accept the feelings … take a slow breath or two … relax your posture … give it a minute or so and let it move away.

6   Notice that once you stop adding frightening thoughts, the fear itself will start to fade – IT ALWAYS DOES.

7   It is important to **practise** these techniques whenever you can in order to get the best from them.

8   Think about any progress you have made, however small. Try to dismiss any negatives. Setbacks will occur from time to time, but these are actually essential to help us learn.

9   Try to describe to yourself what is happening **outside** your body – what is going on around you, in your surroundings or in the distance … take your thoughts away from what your body is telling you and put them outside into the real world.

10   When you feel ready, **slowly** start off again at a relaxed pace. Remind yourself that panic feelings always pass … and that they have passed again, and that you are 'OK'. '**Well done**'.

Self-help approaches

The key steps for the nurse to consider when supporting a patient with mild to moderate anxiety or depression are:

1   information
2   education
3   practice
4   review.

Information

Provide clear information verbally and support this with a good leaflet, booklet, book, audio or video tape. Remember that most patients retain little about what is said in a consultation. Allowing them to take away a resource that they can use at their leisure is not only helpful for the patient, but it can be a huge benefit for their partner or family. Check out the information available from other members of your team, your local community mental health team, health promotion unit and pharmaceutical company representatives. Many of the pharmaceutical companies produce excellent literature for patients which is not designed to promote individual drugs. You will often be able to get hold of this free of charge.

There are also several useful websites. There are a wide variety of patient information leaflets available on the WHO Guide website (www.whoguidemhpcuk.org) which can be printed off. They can also be altered and adapted to fit local circumstances. The guide itself contains a disk giving the whole series of leaflets. Other sources and websites are listed in the Appendix.

Education

This should be done by the nurse initially, but can be backed up by providing further information. Be clear and encourage questions. Identify and correct any erroneous beliefs the patient might have. Repeat explanations and check out that your explanations have been understood. Try to leave no symptom unexplained. It can be helpful to have a tutorial from a GP colleague or perhaps your community mental health nurse (CMHN or CPN) about cause and effect. Use diagrams, pictures and real-life scenarios (as you would when explaining illnesses such as asthma or diabetes).

Practice

Once an explanation has been given, it is then easier to plan an activity, or series of activities for the patient to work on. This could be seen as 'homework', and can be paralleled with the process of learning any new activity (e.g. a language) – it must be practised regularly. Emphasise that there will be 'setbacks'. Setbacks can be seen as opportunities to learn and it must be accepted from the start that they will happen. It can be useful to encourage the patient to keep a 'diary' to note down progress or setbacks.

Review

Never set any homework practice without making sure that you review it. It is important to make a note of the plan/objectives in the patient's notes, and also to note what it is that you are to review. Many patients understandably give up trying if no-one is interested in their progress – so do not forget to check it out and review it with them. In time, you are encouraging the patient to review him/herself ('self-help') and to learn from his/her own observations.

Techniques for 'homework' practice

The following approaches are written AS IF YOU WERE TALKING TO THE PATIENT. Consider how you would word or phrase the following to the patient, and how you would monitor each technique:

- **Self-monitoring:** Monitor your tension and mood levels daily. At the end of each day ask yourself, on a scale of 0–10, how have your tension levels been overall today? Then on the same 0–10 scale, how has your mood been, overall, today? Note these down in a diary. At the end of each week, look at your 'scores' – what do they tell you? Bring your conclusions back to the next appointment. (REASON: to see how moods change and to monitor success and setbacks. It can also help to link feelings with day-to-day events.)
- **Reading up:** Go to your local bookstore or library. Check out some of the titles that relate to your difficulties. If you have a computer and are familiar with browsing the web, try finding further information through reputable sites (e.g. The Royal College of Psychiatrists, MIND, Depression Alliance). (REASON: Understanding symptoms is more than half of the way forward. If you understand the facts, the correct techniques are then logical.)
- **Seeking support:** Do not just deal with this yourself – try to be open with your friends and family. Some people prefer to talk to others who are outside their family and friends. This can be an advantage, since outsiders are not emotionally involved in the situation. There are several self-help groups and organisations that can help. These can often send you information, they may have a local group running in your area, or they may meet regularly and provide support via a group of people who have suffered the same difficulties. Ask your nurse, doctor or health visitor if they know of any organisations that might be able to help. (REASON: Bottling up feelings and worries inside only increases the sense of tension or even hopelessness. Share concerns as well as achievements.)
- **Rest and relaxation:** It is vital to strike a balance between activity and relaxation. The more stressed we are, the more likely we are to have excess energy left – this may feel like tension. Unless you get rid of

this you will simply store it up until you feel like bursting – this can feel like extreme restlessness or agitation, even panic. It is, therefore, important to get plenty of rest; this may simply be learning to have one or more short periods lying down during the day (if you can!), or taking a few slow deep breaths three or four times per day. Such simple activities can profoundly change your blood-gas levels throughout the day, which in turn will help correct your body's chemical balance. If you can, practise some longer sessions of deep relaxation. Audiotapes can be useful for this. (REASON: Relaxation, even short breaks, lowers blood pressure and eases muscle tension. It also balances breathing and produces a sense of heaviness or lightness that is pleasurable.)

- **Exercise:** For some people vigorous exercise provides a sense of achievement and pleasure. Having an excess of tension in the mind or body can produce high levels of natural chemicals such as adrenaline – exercise can get rid of this quickly. For some, however, the opposite is the case – exercise in itself can provoke feelings of breathlessness and tension that may make you feel worse. For this group of people, gentle activity is much more desirable; walking, cycling, swimming or gentle weight training. Try different exercises to see what suits you – but try to take some form of *regular* activity each day, even if it is just for five to ten minutes. Depression may make you lethargic. Introducing gradually increasing exercise into your daily routine will help to overcome the lethargy. (REASON: Exercise helps to dissipate stress hormones and releases endorphins. These natural chemicals improve mood. Your physical health will also benefit and your appetite may improve.)
- **Pampering:** Don't wait for someone else to make you feel good – you don't need 'permission' from others to do this! Treating yourself may not at first feel natural or even 'right' – do not let this stop you. People need treats and simple pleasures. The problem is that many people feel guilty or awkward about pampering themselves. If you feel under-confident, it is harder – but try it, even if it is simply getting yourself a nice magazine, a bar of chocolate, or having a long soak in a bath with aromatherapy oils. Think about what you would like and plan it first. (REASON: Pampering boosts a sense of pleasure and reward, it is a way of 'stroking' ourselves and giving ourselves a feeling of worth. It will also provide a platform to build your self-esteem and allow you to become more assertive.)
- **Problem solving:** Sometimes it is hard to actually identify what is causing you a problem, sometimes you know what it is that is wrong but do not know what to do about it. This technique gives you a

structured way of looking at problems and finding solutions. The steps are as follows.

1 List the problems: Write down all the difficulties that you have (consider relationships, money, work, health etc).
2 Prioritise the problems: Now juggle the list you have made and put them in order of what is the biggest problem, and what is the smallest problem.
3 List all the options: Taking each problem, list down ALL the possible solutions for it – from the silliest to the possible.
4 Pros and Cons: Looking at each of your possible options, make a list of all the 'Pros' (advantages) and 'Cons' (disadvantages).
5 Choose a solution: Now that you have explored all the possible options and looked at all the advantages and disadvantages, choose which one you will try to work on (it might be wise to choose the easiest one first!).
6 Devise a plan: Now work out a step-by-step plan for this option that you have chosen. Break it down into manageable steps, with clear and exact 'instructions' for yourself (consider WHO might help you, HOW and WHEN you will do each step, and any resources you might need). Try to be realistic.
7 Try it out and evaluate: Start your plan, stopping every so often to check how you are doing. If it is going fine, then proceed. If it is going wrong then stop and trace back where it started to go off track – did you miss something? Is there something else you could do to make it work better?
8 If you solved the problem, give yourself a reward and move on to the next problem.

(REASON: To clarify problems and explore options – it is too easy to see one or two possibilities when looking at a difficulty, when in fact there are several possibilities and many options. This is also an approach that can be adopted for future problems.)

Note: Problem solving is done by the patient. The nurse only prompts the steps and helps review progress with the patient. It is important to support and encourage the patient through each stage but it is also important to remember that identified problems must be those perceived by the patient to be problems, not things the nurse believes are problems. Likewise, solutions must be solutions that seem practicable to the patient.

Some problems will not be soluble. For these, the patient will need to learn some coping strategies.

Research into structured problem solving has shown its value as a treatment for severe depression. Mynors-Wallis and colleagues found it to be superior to placebo and as effective as therapeutic doses of amitriptyline.[1] A large European study has also confirmed the efficacy of problem solving and shown its acceptability to patients with depressive illness.[2] This study also seems to suggest that the efficacy of problem solving is not confined to people with major, or severe, depression.

- **Thinking therapy:** Our thoughts are not independent items – each thought produces a range of emotional feelings. To help control our feelings (e.g. anger, guilt, fear) we must learn to take note of our thoughts and try to alter them if they are causing us distress. For instance, when you next feel fear, immediately ask yourself 'What exactly am I thinking just now?' Do not just accept your feelings – learn to question them. Once you start to question your troublesome thoughts, you start to break the vicious circle of Thoughts–Feelings–Behaviours that we can all easily get into:

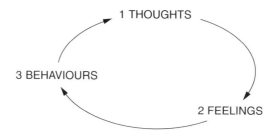

Practise saying to yourself '*STOP!*' when you start to feel bad, rather than allowing the thoughts to continue and repeat, pulling you down further. Stop it in its tracks and question it. Ask yourself if you are telling yourself the truth – is there another thought that would be better for you? This approach is based on a technique that has been used for many decades called 'Cognitive Behavioural Therapy'. (REASON: Repeating 'negative' thoughts produces unpleasant feelings. Learning to stop, block or challenge these thoughts will help to break a pattern of thinking that only makes us feel worse.)

- **Writing and diaries:** It is not always easy, or convenient, to talk to someone about our feelings and worries. Try writing down your thoughts – get it out of your head. You could try keeping a diary of how you feel on a day-to-day basis, and review this (re-read it) once a week to see how you are doing. Write a short conclusion about what you have read. If you have a conflict with a person or an organisation, try writing a letter to that person. In this letter, say exactly what you think – don't hold back, but **DON'T SEND IT!** (REASON: Holding onto troublesome thoughts only causes more misery and emotional pain. Writing them down gets them out, allows us to examine them at a later time, and helps us to learn more about ourselves through time. It can also help us to come to a conclusion about the person or organisation that has caused us so much strife. Alternatively try writing poetry, even if you have never done it before.)
- **Talking and sharing:** Sometimes simply sharing our worries with another person eases the discomfort that it causes. We do not all have people in our lives that we feel we can trust and be open with, but sharing a problem need not mean talking about it (although this is preferable) – some people write their worries (*see* above), some pray, some draw or paint, while some meditate. There are many ways to 'dilute' our worries, but it is important that we try not to hold onto all of our emotional pain without sharing some of it. Sometimes it is better to talk to someone outside of our circle of friends and family, and this might mean seeing a counsellor or specialist. (REASON: Talking helps us put a perspective on our difficulties. It can help us find new ways of dealing with the problems and help us to understand why we react to some things the way we do. It may allow us to see things from a different angle.)

The primary care nurse already has the skills required to carry through many of the above approaches. They do not require specialist training. But nurses may need to recognise the skills that they already have and are presently using on a day-to-day basis – listening, evaluating, monitoring, using basic counselling skills, structured action planning. These are transferable skills. Many nurses have the interest and confidence to apply them to a wide variety of situations. Nurses are usually very good at explaining illnesses and providing good health promotion to patients. Promoting mental health is no different.

Summary of steps

1   To help the person acknowledge their stress, anxiety or depression.
2   To explain what stress is – including common signs and symptoms.
3   Explain how the biological changes produce both physical *and* emotional symptoms. Try to clarify the links between the symptoms and what is going on in their life, past and present.
4   Explain clearly each of the individual symptoms that the person presents with, clarifying HOW this symptom is actually produced.
5   Tailor a regime of exercise/relaxation to fit the symptoms, explaining again why these exercises are appropriate. A clear programme of WHEN to do these exercises and for HOW LONG for should be negotiated.
6   Agree a follow-up session, clarifying exactly what is expected in terms of a) what the patient should be practising (and perhaps how to monitor and record progress), and b) what you as a nurse will be looking at on the next appointment, e.g. reviewing progress and 'setbacks', providing further written information, going through an explanation of the symptoms again (do this repeatedly to make sure that the patient moves towards a greater understanding, and less fear of, the symptoms). Follow-up sessions are also useful times to reassess.

A useful resource to help your knowledge and understanding about stress and anxiety could be your CMHN (CPN) or practice counsellor. Your own GPs may be the first place to start in terms of organising a tutorial within the practice, and do not forget that some of the pharmaceutical representatives may have this as their specialist subject and may be willing to organise a training event and provide practical resources.

Being 'stress free' is not only unrealistic in this modern world, it is also an impossibility! But we all need to understand and manage our stress so that it doesn't become *DIS*tress. No-one is immune from 'catching' it, including NHS staff. All the techniques described in this chapter can be used by nurses for themselves.

Look after yourself as well as your patients and clients.

References

1   Mynors-Wallis LM, Gath DH, Lloyd-Thomas AR *et al.* (1995) Randomised controlled trial comparing problem solving treatment with amitriptyline and placebo for major depression in primary care. *BMJ.* **310**: 441–5.

2 Dowrick C, Dunn G, Ayuso-Mateos JL *et al.* and the Outcomes of Depression International Network (ODIN) Group (2000) Problem solving treatment and group psychoeducation for depression: multicentre randomised controlled trial. *BMJ.* **321**: 1–6.

Further reading

Butler G and Hope T (1999) *Manage Your Mind.* Oxford University Press, New York.

CHAPTER FOUR

Alcohol and illegal drugs

Jim Barnard and Simon Morton

Introduction

Primary care is often seen by commissioners and policy makers as the preferred venue for the screening and, in many cases, the treatment of drug and alcohol problems.[1,2] There are many reasons for this. In terms of alcohol, general practice is the most likely place for a patient with an undiagnosed drug and alcohol problem to present, often with a separate, but related, condition. In general practice the totality of health need can be addressed and the patient history and circumstances are usually better known. Treatment in primary care with the support of a specialist worker is often viewed as the preferred option. The same is true for the treatment of drug users particularly since specialist services, who offer long-term treatment, cannot cope with providing all the care for all the patients. The option of 'shared care' is attractive in terms of increasing the capacity to deal with a larger number of patients. Primary care itself is often resistant to such arrangements partly because it is seen as yet another thing that an over-stretched service has to deal with but also that they do not have the knowledge or the time to effectively deal with such patients. Furthermore, these patients, particularly drug users, are often viewed as a 'nuisance' in that they present unwanted management problems.[3,4] This chapter aims to provide some essential knowledge around this issue for those working in primary care as well as laying out effective patient management tools.

Overview of substance misuse

It is important to realise that substance misuse is not a modern phenomenon. There is evidence going back to 5000 BC that the Sumerians were using opium.[5] The first alcohol licensing system existed in Babylon in 1770 BC, and the earliest reference to cannabis intoxication is about 2000 BC. The Delphic Oracle in Greece used to get her hallucinations from sniffing gases emanating from a crevice in the rocks. More recently Hogarth's Gin Alley showed the damage caused to society by alcohol in the 18th century. Controls on substance use are also not new. In the later middle ages the death penalty existed in both Germany and part of the Ottoman Empire for coffee drinking and also in Germany for smoking tobacco. This section will lay out some information on the most commonly used drugs in society at the present time.

Drugs used for intoxication can be broadly split into three categories:

- depressants of the central nervous system that slow down and shut down bodily functions
- stimulants of the central nervous system that speed up and enhance bodily functions
- hallucinogens which do neither but alter the user's perception of the world around them.

Depressants of the central nervous system

These include drugs such as heroin and all opiates, alcohol, benzodiazepine tranquillisers, solvents and, to a partial extent, cannabis. These drugs sedate and slow down performance. They are the drugs most associated with causing a physical illness on withdrawal as well as the psychological craving and obsession which they share with the stimulants. They are also the drugs most associated with fatal overdose, particularly opiates and alcohol. Death is by respiratory failure caused by the system being so depressed that it ceases to function.

They are also the most dangerous drugs to take in combination. Mixing two or three depressants together is much more likely to result in serious complications than one on its own. Mixing a depressant and a stimulant to some extent cancels itself out and a combination of stimulants, while dangerous, is much less likely to be fatal. The depressants are also the drugs which have the best-researched treatment options and are the most likely to be encountered in primary care.

Alcohol

This is obviously a very popular drug. It is a depressant that can be fatal in overdose (alcohol poisoning) and can cause physical and psychological dependency. The withdrawal syndrome (unlike heroin withdrawal) is potentially fatal and thus a severely dependent individual should not stop drinking abruptly without medication. Drinking above the safe limits (3–4 units a day for men and 2–3 units a day for women) can cause a whole range of physical and mental health problems. Drinking is also associated with violent behaviour and child protection issues.

Treatment

Early intervention is important, as it is associated with better outcomes. Primary care is the ideal setting for this. It is useful for all patients to be asked about their drinking levels. General signs of excessive alcohol usage can include:

- repeated physical evidence (e.g. smell, discarded bottles/cans etc)
- regular falls/accidents
- poor nutrition
- social isolation/active social life
- self-neglect
- signs of dependence (tremor, craving)
- financial problems
- employment problems
- depression
- alcohol-related health problems (too many to list).

(*See also* Chapter 2 – CAGE Questionnaire.)

Once an alcohol problem is suspected, before proceeding it may be best to discuss approaches with a colleague or supervisor. It is usually better to discuss the matter directly with the person in a matter of fact way without appearing to judge or lecture. It is best to concentrate on observed behaviour rather than giving an opinion, for instance 'I can't help noticing you are spending most of your money on drink rather than food' as opposed to 'I think you're an alcoholic'. Fear of a negative response should not be a reason not to raise the issue.

If the problem is of a less severe nature it can be dealt with in primary care through the use of practical approaches such as drink diaries and action plans to reduce the amount consumed. In moderate to severe cases a specialist assessment is probably necessary. There is usually a specialist alcohol service in every area that can provide this. Depending on local circumstances, on-going treatment may be conducted by specialists or by shared care between the specialist service and primary care. Medical treatment in the more severe cases is usually centred around the prescribing of chlordiazepoxide (Librium) for the withdrawal phase and acamprosate (Campral) or disulfuram (Antabuse) for relapse prevention, but social support and psychosocial interventions are more important especially when it comes to relapse prevention.

Possibly the group of people whose alcohol problems are least likely to be identified are older people. One survey found that GPs had a zero rate of detection of alcohol problems in older women.[6] Another survey found that whilst hospital admissions directly for alcohol-related problems among those over 65 were running at 13.3% of the total, older people represented less than 2% of the treatment population for alcohol problems.[7] This is compounded by the fact that alcohol has a disproportionately serious effect on older people with safe drinking levels estimated to be one unit a day.[8] As well as the above checklist for identification, issues such as confusion and incontinence are more likely to be exacerbated in older drinkers. Older people may be less likely to admit to an alcohol problem due to the social stigma and are less likely to feel pressure to address it from family members or employers. However, older people have more contact with the health service in general and primary care in particular so it is important that professionals working in primary care do not turn a blind eye to this issue.

Opiates/heroin

Heroin (diamorphine) is an extremely effective painkiller and is used widely in terminal care and heart disease. It is also a drug of misuse from which physical dependency can develop quite quickly. It is known colloquially as *smack*, *skag*, *h*, *gear* or *horse* (among others) and is either smoked (*chasing*) or injected (*fixing*, *cranking*). It works as a very effective emotional painkiller with users reporting that they feel like they are wrapped in cotton wool. Opiate dependency is often associated with crime to feed the habit with up to £300–£400 a week needing to be raised. The withdrawal syndrome is typified by severe flu type symptoms as well as insomnia. The temptation to use again is very strong as the user knows that one hit will make them feel better. Interestingly it does not have very many side effects, the main ones being constipation and reduced sex drive. The main dangers are overdose (potentially fatal), which can occur at doses close to the psychoactive dose, and diseases contracted from the use of contaminated injecting equipment. Apart from heroin the main opiates used are methadone, morphine, dihydrocodeine, buprenorphine and pethedine.

Treatment

Treatment for opiate dependency is long established and dates back to the Rolleston report of 1926, which stated that doctors could prescribe heroin to *bona fide addicts*. This system is broadly still in place with the preferred substitute drug being methadone, a long-acting synthetic opioid which produces less of a high and which, it is argued, encourages greater stability in the patient's life. Increasingly, with the rise in opiate dependency, primary care is being asked to take a role in the treatment of these patients. This is usually in partnership with a specialist treatment provider in what is known as a shared care arrangement. This involves the GP writing the prescription working closely with a drug worker. One of the advantages of these arrangements is that it gives drug users better access to general medical services. Injecting drug users have specific health needs, particularly hepatitis C which has infected a very high proportion of users. Users should be offered testing for this alongside counselling and advice. Intravenous drug users should also be offered hepatitis B vaccination if not already infected. HIV testing and pre- and post-test counselling should also be offered. There is a whole range of problems associated with injecting (e.g. deep vein thrombosis, abscesses, endocarditis) which will need to be monitored.

Management

The fear of violence, abuse or disruption by drug users to staff or other patients in the surgery is common among primary care workers. In numerous surveys of GPs, it is the anticipation of these sorts of problems which is often cited as a reason for not wanting to treat drug users. In fact, despite the relative insecurity of the primary care setting, these individuals can be managed successfully by the primary care team. Perhaps the most important factor in promoting successful management of this patient group is the consistency of approach from the team as a whole. One study suggests that it is not the presence of drug using patients *per se* which is the problem, but the extent to which there is a clarity and consistency of approach (or lack of one) in the practice.[9]

In order to ensure consistency, a practice policy can be useful.[10] Both clinical staff who are not GPs and non-clinical staff play important roles in managing drug users in the practice and, although GPs may be ultimately clinically responsible, involving the wider team in consultation and development of policies will pay dividends. Policies might cover, for example, appointments, prescriptions and unacceptable behaviour, and once drawn up can be reviewed and audited. A copy of the policy can be given to and explained to patients.

A policy for temporary residents and urgent, necessary patients is particularly important. Some drug users or those trying to obtain drugs to sell often register in this way in order to obtain drugs, such as opiates and benzodiazepines, quickly. They are often not seeking treatment but a quick 'score' and do not usually present to specialist agencies if referred. If prescribed for, it may cause ongoing disruption in the surgery and contribute to the wider problems within the community. It can be useful to have a policy, backed up by a leaflet, which can be given to all patients registering temporarily or urgently stating that the following drugs will not be prescribed and referring requests back to the permanent GP or to the specialist service. The issue of benzodiazepines is worth exploring in some detail within the practice team. A practice that wished to make a start on tackling local community drug problems could do worse than beginning with the problems posed by benzodiazepines.

Good communication, both within the team and with outside agencies, though obvious, is vital. It will be useful to know the number of the local drug service and the name, if there is one, of the service's nominated liaison worker. 'Shared care' for drug users is becoming increasingly widespread and drug services generally put a premium on supporting and advising GPs and primary care team staff.

Finally, having a good basic understanding of the drugs themselves will go a long way to helping all staff feel more confident when talking to a drug-using patient. Local health promotion units and community drug teams will have details of drug awareness courses that may run regularly.

Benzodiazepines

First formulated in the late 1950s and heralded as the safe alternative to barbiturates, benzodiazepine tranquillisers are meant to be prescribed either for anxiety or insomnia. Whilst not being as dangerous as barbiturates in overdose or withdrawal they have still proved to be extremely problematic drugs. Dependency forms easily and the withdrawal syndrome is typified by extreme brain hyperactivity where the individual often feels they are 'going mad'. Fits are also reported. As a result of this they are now recommended to be prescribed for two weeks only. They have also replaced barbiturates on the illegal market with users taking them, sometimes by crushing and injecting, to get very heavily intoxicated to the extent that they will have no memory of events. Up to 25% of users in this state become physically aggressive, and intoxication is typified by wild disinhibition. There are serious possibilities of both violent and acquisitive crime taking place. Benzodiazepines are often mixed with alcohol to heighten the effect. The most popular drugs in the illegal market are diazepam (diazzies), temazepam (temazzies) and nitrazepam (moggies). As well as the illegal usage there are probably many hundreds of thousands of people who are therapeutically dependent on these drugs.

Treatment

There is no evidence that prescribing benzodiazepines to illegal drug users reduces harm to themselves or society, rather the opposite. Due to the severe withdrawal syndrome if someone is known to be dependent, a reducing prescription can sometimes be justified but only with specialist advice. Patients who are therapeutically dependent should be given support to try and come off and may need a specialist referral or referral to a support group. Patients in this group who do succeed in coming off usually report that their quality of life is greatly enhanced. Benzodiazepines (along with alcohol) are probably responsible for a large amount of disruption and aggression in general practice settings and arguments over prescriptions are even more common than with drugs such as methadone. They are, however, the drug of choice for alcohol detoxification (*see* p. 54, Librium).

Solvents

These encompass a range of household products, most famously glue and aerosols. The vapours are inhaled and the user becomes intoxicated in a way similar to alcohol. However, repeated sniffing can cause hallucinations which are often sought by users. Until the early 1990s they were the biggest killers of children under 16. Although deaths are no longer at this level they are still significant. Death is usually from suffocation (on polythene bag) or through freezing of the throat by spraying directly into the mouth. Fortunately most users grow out of the habit by their mid-teens as it is not viewed as a socially acceptable form of behaviour even in drug using circles (hence there are no slang terms for solvents). However those that do persist are often some of the most damaged individuals in society and become completely socially isolated sniffing alone with no social circle. In cases of adolescent experimentation, providing information and advice may be enough, but with persistent use a specialist referral will be necessary.

Cannabis

This is the most commonly used illegal drug about which much has been written elsewhere. It has more slang terms than any other drug (most commonly *puff*, *draw*, *weed*). It has an effect that is part depressant, part hallucinogen and mildly stimulant due to the wide variety of active chemicals in it. As a result it is not associated with overdose like the other depressants and does not have a physical withdrawal syndrome of the nature of alcohol, benzodiazepines or heroin. Many people do become psychologically dependent and this can affect their quality of life. It can also cause relapse in people with psychotic illnesses. Indeed, extreme paranoia whilst intoxicated is a reaction commonly reported by users. Many mental health workers report it as the most problematic drug for their client group. Treatment is usually the same as for a mild alcohol problem (*see* p. 54) with joint diaries replacing drink diaries. Occasionally there may be a need for a specialist referral especially where there are mental health issues. It is worth noticing that the majority of users of other drugs will also be using cannabis but may not regard this as a problem.

Stimulants of the central nervous system

These are drugs that make the user feel more confident and alert and suppress sleep and appetite. They include drugs such as cocaine, amphetamine, nicotine and caffeine. Whilst not creating a physical withdrawal like some depressants the psychological distress of abstinence can in some cases be so severe as to feel physical. One only has to look at the difficulty smokers have in giving up to realise how powerful this can be.

Cocaine and amphetamine

In some respects the effects of cocaine (*coke, charlie, snow*) and amphetamine (*speed, whizz, billy, sulphate*) are similar. Both are powerful stimulants with cocaine being short acting (effects lasting half an hour if sniffed and 15 minutes if injected) and amphetamine long acting (lasting up to 8 hours if sniffed or swallowed). If used occasionally and the body and mind are allowed time to recover then long-term problems are rare. If used daily in large amounts, then a range of problems can develop such as paranoia, weight loss, insomnia, aggression and in some cases temporary psychosis. In these cases withdrawal from the drug can trigger a clinical depression as well as an accompanying extreme tiredness and appetite loss. In recent years a smokeable version of cocaine (*crack*) has appeared which provides an 8–10 minute high of greater intensity than cocaine but with resultant greater cravings and withdrawal symptoms. The use of this drug on the street drug-using scene has resulted in habits of over £1000 a week in many cases, which has even greater implications for the individual and society than a heroin habit.

Stimulant users do not often present to primary care, as there is no recognised medical treatment apart perhaps from the use of SSRI antidepressants in abstinent patients. However, a sympathetic, non-medical response in primary care has been found to be appreciated by stimulant users. Innovative, non-medical services have started to develop and it is worth enquiring as to whether there is one in the local area. In severe cases a specialist referral is necessary.

Hallucinogens

These include drugs such as LSD, magic mushrooms and Ecstasy. Pure hallucinogens such as LSD (*acid, trips*) and mushrooms (*mushies*) send the user on an 8–12 hour 'trip' during which the user perceives the world in a different way and may experience hallucinations and other perceptual distortions. This can be a very rewarding experience for some, for others a bad trip can lead to severe psychological distress and even trigger latent mental disorders. These drugs are not dependency forming as the effects disappear if taken for more than a few days in succession and a break is necessary to experience them again. Someone who has had a bad trip is unlikely to repeat the experience so the best treatment is talking through the experience and reassuring the user that they will recover in time. In cases of severe distress, a specialist (possibly mental health) referral is necessary.

Ecstasy

Ecstasy has hit the headlines due to many high profile deaths. It in fact kills about eight people a year, far fewer than all the depressant drugs (except cannabis). Death is usually by heat stroke aggravated by the setting in which the drug is taken (clubs and raves). In the case of Leah Betts, probably the most high profile case, death was due to drinking too much water to compensate for the overheating, this combined with the anti-diuretic effects of the drug meant that she died of too much water flooding the brain. Ecstasy is a partial stimulant related to amphetamine with mild hallucinogenic qualities. It is much milder than LSD so a bad trip is uncommon and less serious. It is not often used dependently but its problems and treatment would be similar to the stimulants. Long-term use has also been reported to cause depression, perhaps due to reducing serotonin levels.

Dual diagnosis

The term 'dual diagnosis' in the substance misuse field refers to the co-existence of mental health problems and problematic drug or alcohol use, and indicates a close relationship between the respective conditions. However, the growing significance of 'polydrug use' (the combined use of substances including alcohol) and the complex causal relationship between mental health problems and substance misuse mean that the term 'co-morbidity' might be more useful.

People with mental health problems are likely to be no different than the general population in their exposure to and use of substances. Drugs such as amphetamine and cocaine can precipitate psychotic reactions, and studies have shown an increasing prevalence of use in the population. Other drugs such as cannabis, alcohol, ecstasy and LSD are also used and, like the stimulant drugs, can also worsen existing symptoms of mental disorders and bring about relapse in recurrent conditions. Interestingly, some drugs like heroin or methadone may alleviate some of the symptoms of psychotic conditions and may be used as a kind of self-medication. However, while opiates have been used by probably only 1% of society, use of alcohol and cannabis is so widespread and potentially risky to mental health that it is a serious cause for concern.

Studies of 'dual diagnosis' or 'co-morbid' patients have repeatedly shown that they tend to have more frequent hospitalisations; greater use of emergency services; greater likelihood of homelessness; greater propensity to violent or unsociable behaviour; increased vulnerability to suicide; enhanced health risks (e.g. HIV, poor eating habits, liver damage); and poorer compliance with treatment and medication. While this catalogue of need is striking, these individuals are further handicapped by the difficulty they have in receiving treatment because psychiatric services and drug services sometimes regard these people as each other's responsibility.

Primary care professionals should regularly screen for, and be able to provide, brief interventions for anxiety and mood disorders in patients using substances. Patients with more severe cases of 'dual diagnosis' or 'co-morbidity' will usually need a specialist referral. Many of these individuals will have complex needs requiring social services and housing agencies to provide input alongside primary care and medical services. They may also be receiving input on a statutory basis from agencies such as the probation service. Consequently, local arrangements which promote an integrated, multidisciplinary approach will provide the best way of ensuring appropriate services to this difficult to engage patient group.

Conclusion

Problems around drugs and alcohol are endemic in the UK at the present time. It is thus a fact that all primary care professions will need to deal with these issues at some level. The good news is that it is not as scary a subject as the media sometimes portrays and with enough knowledge and confidence primary care is well equipped to deal appropriately with anyone presenting there.

References

1 DoH (1995) *Reviewed Shared Care Arrangements for Drug Misusers.* Executive Letter EL (95) 114. DoH, London.

2 DoH (1999) *Drug Misuse and Dependence: guidelines on clinical management.* The Stationery Office, London.

3 Greenwood J (1992) Persuading general practitioners to prescribe: good husbandry or a recipe for chaos? *Br J Addic.* **87**: 567–75.

4 Barnard J and Higson J (1999) Caring and sharing: modelling successful shared care. *Druglink.* **Jan/Feb**.

5 Smith I (1999) *History of drugs and drug controls.* Trafford Substance Misuse Service. Unpublished.

6 Ward M (1997) *Alcohol and Older People: a neglected area.* A literature review. Health Education Authority, London.

7 Timms L and Barnard J (1997) *Alcohol Related Ill-health in Older People: needs assessment report.* Joint Commissioning Board for Substance Misuse, Southampton and South West Hampshire. Southampton and South West Hampshire Health Authority.

8 Alcohol Concern (1995) *Alcohol and Older People.* Information Unit factsheet.

9 Hawkes R and Cyster R (1998) *The Shared Care of Drug Users in Calderdale and Kirklees.* RSDC, Leeds.

10 Beaumont B (ed.) (1997) *Care of Drug Users in General Practice.* Radcliffe Medical Press, Oxford.

Further reading

Beaumont B (ed.) (1997) *Care of Drug Users in General Practice.* Radcliffe Medical Press, Oxford.

Harrison L (1996) *Alcohol Problems in the Community.* Routledge, London.

ISDD (Drugscope) (1999) *Drug Abuse Briefing.* ISDD, London.

Preston A (1996) *The Methadone Briefing.* ISDD, London.

Tyler A (1995) *Street Drugs.* Hodder & Stoughton, London.

Ward M and Goodman C (1995) *Alcohol Problems in Old Age: a practical guide to helping older people with alcohol problems* (2e). Wynne Howard Publishing, London.

CHAPTER FIVE

Eating disorders

Elizabeth Armstrong

Introduction

The role of primary care teams in the treatment of people with eating disorders is not very clear though it is a requirement that teams should have a protocol under the National Service Framework for Mental Health (Standard 2). Casey suggested that most people with eating disorders would be referred for specialist help and that there was therefore a limited role for the GP.[1] Goldberg and Gourney agreed that people with severe eating disorders required referral, but that there was a role for primary care teams in mild disorders.[2]

This role should probably concentrate on recognition as early as possible, though this can be difficult, and in early intervention to minimise consequent physical and emotional damage. Whether or not early intervention is likely to prevent progression to more serious disorders, which have poor prognosis, may be open to question and requires much more research at primary care level.

What are eating disorders?

The two most common of these disorders are anorexia nervosa and bulimia nervosa. The Eating Disorders Association estimates that each GP list of approximately 2000 patients will include:

- 1–2 patients with anorexia
- 18 patients with bulimia

- 5–10% of adolescent girls who are using weight reduction techniques other than dieting, for example vomiting, diuretic misuse or excessive exercising.

Both anorexia and bulimia are characterised by secrecy and it has been suggested that they may lead to considerable undiagnosed morbidity and mortality because many sufferers do not seek medical help.[3,4]

Anorexia and bulimia are both more common amongst women and young girls than amongst men. Both conditions tend to develop between the ages of 15 and 25, though they can occur at any age. The age of onset of anorexia is commonly about 16 in girls though possibly earlier in boys.[1] Bulimia is rare before age 13 but usually presents at around age 25. It is also suggested that many patients with bulimia will have met the criteria for anorexia at some time in their lives. Anorexia is said to be associated particularly with middle and upper socioeconomic groups; bulimia crosses all groups equally. Both conditions are said to be less common in ethnic minority groups than in the indigenous white population.

The role of the media, particularly women's magazines, in promoting thinness as the ideal for women, has been much criticised for encouraging a climate in which eating disorders may become more prevalent. Women in occupations where it is seen as necessary to control weight and maintain fitness, such as dancers, models, actresses and athletes may be at particular risk. Eating disorders may develop in response to the pressures young people experience in puberty and growing up.

Peate introduces a note of caution.[5] Though eating disorders may be more common in women, he believes that these conditions are often overlooked in men and that the illness may be well established and cause much long-term suffering before treatment is offered. He quotes research suggesting that up to 20% of males suffering from eating disorders are gay, which is twice the estimated proportion of gay men in the population. This may help to reinforce the belief that gender and sexuality issues are important in eating disorders, though the exact way in which the conditions are influenced is unclear.

People with anorexia have not lost their appetite. They are often frightened to eat. Eating means putting on weight, growing, becoming adult. Starving oneself is a way of staying in control, of remaining a child, of not having to face the adult world.

In bulimia, the conflict may be between putting on weight, which is undesirable, and an intense desire to eat. Vomiting may seem the only way to eat and still avoid getting fat. The common factor in both conditions is the need to maintain control over food and body.[6] Peate suggests that a common trigger for both men and women may be bullying.[5]

There is some indication that eating disorders may run in families, though the mechanism is not clear. There is a widespread belief that eating disorders are more common in women from families which are rigid and over-protective, or where there might be unrealistically high expectations. There may also be associations with parental alcohol misuse or childhood sexual abuse.

It may in fact be the case that there are general associations between family dysfunction and psychological disorders, rather than with specific conditions.[7] A recent study has looked at the association between childhood sexual abuse and depression.[8] This study concluded that there was an association, but that depression was most likely to occur in women who had suffered severe childhood sexual abuse (defined as penetration or attempted penetration). Other studies have found associations between severe childhood sexual abuse and antisocial behaviour, suicidal behaviour and drug and alcohol misuse amongst adolescents.[9,10]

Recognition

The *WHO Guide to Mental Health in Primary Care* does not separate out anorexia and bulimia. Patients may use binge eating or extreme weight control measures such as self-induced vomiting, excessive consumption of diet pills or laxatives at different times. People with either condition may come to the notice of the primary care team because of physical disorders such as amenorrhoea, fits or cardiac arrhythmias which require monitoring and treatment. Alternatively, family members may ask for help because of the patient's loss of weight, refusal to eat, vomiting or amenorrhoea. Raphael suggests that requests for repeat prescriptions for laxatives, diuretics or appetite suppressants should be questioned.[7]

The diagnostic features of eating disorders are:

- unreasonable fear of being fat or overweight
- extensive efforts to control weight, for example, strict dieting, vomiting, use of purgatives, excessive exercise
- denial that weight or eating habits are a problem
- low mood, anxiety, irritability
- obsessional symptoms

- relationship difficulties
- increasing withdrawal
- school or work problems.

People with anorexia may show:

- severe dieting despite very low body weight
- distorted body image – that is an unreasonable belief of being over-weight despite evidence to the contrary
- amenorrhoea.

Other signs may include: excessive exercising; wearing baggy clothes; increasing isolation and loss of friends; moodiness; perfectionism and obsessional, ritualistic behaviour especially about food and calories; feeling cold with poor circulation and a growth of downy hair all over the body.

People with bulimia may show:

- binge eating – eating large amounts of food in a few hours
- purging – attempts to eliminate food by self-induced vomiting or use of diuretics or laxatives.

Other signs may include: disappearing to the lavatory after meals in order to get rid of food eaten; secretive behaviour; feeling out of control, helpless and lonely; mood swings; sore throat and erosion of tooth enamel caused by vomiting; dehydration and poor skin condition; 'hamster' cheeks caused by enlarged salivary glands from vomiting; lethargy.

Depression may be present in patients with either anorexia or bulimia and there may be associated problems of alcohol or drug misuse.

It is important that patients with eating disorders are recognised early. Mild eating disorders are easier to treat, though even in these cases, a proportion of sufferers will become chronic. The prognosis for severe eating disorders is not good.

Assessment

It can be very difficult to recognise the early signs of eating disorders, but Raphael suggests that particular attention should be paid, in general practice settings, to young women who present frequently with non-specific menstrual problems, abdominal or gynaecological symptoms.[7] School nurses will also have a role to play in early recognition, and also in providing appropriate education about nutrition and dieting.

Some suitable opening questions might be:

- How much exercise do you do? (Is this more than your friends?)
- Are you happy with your weight?
- Do you diet?
- Do you feel in control of your eating?
- Do you ever find you can't stop eating when you want to?
- Do you ever fast for whole days at a time?

Other possible questions include:

- Do you always want to eat less than other people in your family (or your friends)?
- Are you always counting calories?
- Are you worried about the shape of your body or your weight?
- Do you like to eat alone?

If these questions give rise to concern, then more direct questions may be needed, for example:

- When was your last period?
- Do you ever vomit, use laxatives or diuretics? If so, how much and when?
- Do you ever binge? How often and what do you eat?
- Have you noticed any weakness in your muscles? What about climbing the stairs?
- What is your sleep like?
- Have you fainted or had dizzy spells?

(Questions adapted from Raphael (1996) and *Eating Disorders: a guide for primary care*, The Eating Disorders Association.)

Before a diagnosis of an eating disorder can be made, physical conditions which can lead to weight loss must be excluded. Blood chemistry estimations will be needed, particularly urea and electrolytes. A body mass index

(BMI) of less than $13.5 \, \text{kg/m}^2$ is an indication for urgent referral to a service with expertise in eating disorders.

Treatment

People with mild eating disorders can often be effectively treated in primary care, once they have been recognised. For disorders that have been present for some time, specialist help is likely to be needed. Even with prompt treatment, a proportion of people with mild eating disorders will develop chronic conditions.

The first step in treatment is to help the person acknowledge that they have a problem and to offer support. Education about nutrition, weight and dieting may be helpful. Back-up written material should be available for both patient and family and the advice and support of a dietician may be useful.

In anorexia, a food diary may be used to set and monitor goals for weight gain. Any goals must be realistic and should be negotiated and agreed with the patient. It may take many months to reach a 'normal' weight, but provided that the patient's weight does not go down to a dangerous level, the process must not be rushed. A supportive family member may be able to help. An experienced practice counsellor may be able to provide psychological therapies to tackle underlying problems. There is currently no evidence that drug therapy is effective in anorexia, though co-existing depression may respond to antidepressants.

Food diaries can also be useful in bulimia. It may be possible to help patients recognise their triggers for binge eating and then to devise alternative strategies for dealing with them. As with anorexia, counselling may be helpful. Antidepressants may also have a place in reducing bingeing and vomiting but concordance may be poor.

Family therapy may be helpful for patients with anorexia. Cognitive behavioural therapy may be effective in either condition. Self-help approaches may be particularly useful in bulimia. The Eating Disorders Association (EDA) runs a 10-week telephone support programme for patients who are under the supervision of a GP. The programme aims to help patients re-establish a normal eating pattern by encouraging the patient to agree to:

- eat three regular meals a day
- keep a diary to record food and feelings

- make a weekly phone call to an EDA counsellor for 45 minutes of counselling
- send the diary to the counsellor each week
- attend a GP surgery at an agreed time each week to be weighed – weight to be recorded in the diary
- make follow-up calls to the counsellor after the programme.

Patients using this programme must be normal weight for height and must not be abusing drugs or alcohol.

The Eating Disorders Association also has a network of self-help groups throughout the country. Self-help groups are likely to include greater numbers of women. They may therefore be seen as less appropriate for men. Telephone help lines may be more acceptable.

Urgent referral to specialist services is required if body mass index is too low, or if the following are present:

- potassium levels are less than 2.5 mmol/l
- severe bone marrow dysfunction with loss of platelets
- evidence of proximal myopathy
- significant gastrointestinal symptoms from repeated vomiting, e.g. blood in vomit
- significant suicide risk
- other complicating factors, e.g. drug or alcohol misuse.

Patients may need to be referred for assessment on a less urgent basis if there is lack of progress using primary care measures as above. Specialist services for patients with eating disorders may be patchy throughout the country but the requirements of the National Service Framework for Mental Health may give impetus to a move for better access.

Conclusion

Research into eating disorders at primary care level seems sparse and there is little acknowledgement in the nursing literature that primary care nurses may have a role to play. Key issues appear to be awareness of the possibilities of these conditions in young people who are losing weight and exercising excessively. Early intervention is likely to be more effective than treatment that is started when the condition has become well established.

References

1   Casey PR (1993) *A Guide to Psychiatry in Primary Care* (Chapter 14). Wrightson Biomedical Publishing, Petersfield.

2   Goldberg D and Gournay K (1997) *The General Practitioner, the Psychiatrist and the Burden of Mental Health Care.* Maudsley discussion paper No. 1. Institute of Psychiatry, London.

3   Perry M (2000) Eating disorders (part 1). *Practice Nursing.* **11**(8): 8–12.

4   Perry M (2000) Eating disorders (part 2). *Practice Nursing.* **11**(9): 17–19.

5   Peate I (2001) Male eating disorders. *Practice Nursing.* **12**(3): 116–18.

6   Duker M and Slade R (1988) *Anorexia Nervosa and Bulimia: how to help.* Open University Press, Milton Keynes.

7   Raphael F (1996) The prevention of eating disorders. In: T Kendrick, A Tylee and P Freeling (eds) *The Prevention of Mental Illness in Primary Care.* Cambridge University Press, Cambridge.

8   Cheasty M, Clare AW and Collins C (1998) Relation between sexual abuse in childhood and adult depression: case control study. *BMJ.* **316**: 198–202.

9   Bensley LS, Van Eenwyk J, Spieker SJ *et al.* (1999) Self-reported abuse history and adolescent problem behaviours. 1. Antisocial and suicidal behaviours. *J Adolesc Health.* **24**(3): 163–72.

10 Bensley LS, Spieker SJ, Van Eenwyk J *et al.* (1999) Self-reported abuse history and adolescent problem behaviours. 2. Alcohol and drug use. *J Adolesc Health.* **24**(3): 173–80.

CHAPTER SIX

Serious mental illness in primary care

Heather Raistrick and Elizabeth Armstrong

Introduction

The majority of patients with severe and enduring mental health problems are registered with a general practitioner. People who suffer long-term mental health problems have poor access to primary healthcare for a variety of reasons which might include lack of social skills and reduced mobility. With these factors in mind they are also more vulnerable to physical health problems. Strathdee and Kendrick point out that schizophrenia is associated with increased death rates from cardiovascular and respiratory diseases, some of which are preventable.[1] They also quote studies showing that a high proportion of people with schizophrenia have unmet physical health needs.

There are many definitions of severe and enduring mental illness. One of the most commonly used is that of Kendrick who defines a person with long-term mental illness as someone who for two or more years has been disabled by impaired social behaviour as a consequence of mental illness.[2] Disability is the defining criterion; the patient being unable to fulfil one of four roles:

- holding down a job
- self-care and personal hygiene
- performing necessary domestic chores
- participating in recreational activities.

The National Service Framework for Mental Health sets out clear standards for people who suffer from a mental illness. Those who suffer from a severe and enduring mental illness usually receive care from specialist services. Specialist services are being encouraged to work in partnership with social care, the independent sector and agencies that provide housing, training and employment. Primary care organisations are actively being encouraged to participate in this package of care.

Primary care organisations are the designated lead organisations for Standards 2 and 3 of the framework. The aim of these standards is to deliver better primary mental health care, and to ensure consistent advice and help for people with mental health needs, including primary care services for individuals with severe mental illness. The framework gives two alternative definitions of severe mental illness, but these are not inconsistent with that of Kendrick.

Severe mental illness

In practice, the most common forms of severe mental illness are schizophrenia, bipolar disorder and puerperal psychosis. It is important to remember that patients with very severe depression may be considerably disabled by their condition and are likely to fall into this category. Severe mental illness is not confined to those illnesses often described as 'psychoses'.

Acute psychosis

Psychosis is defined in the *Collins English Dictionary* as any severe mental disorder in which the individual's contact with reality becomes highly distorted. Medically, these conditions include schizophrenia and other illnesses which present in similar ways. Patients' experiences will be outside the normal range, and may include:

- hallucinations, which may be visual or auditory
- strange beliefs or fears
- apprehension, confusion
- perceptual changes.

People with psychoses may not recognise that they are ill or that their experiences are part of an illness. Families may ask for help with behaviour changes that cannot be explained, including strange or frightening behaviour (e.g. withdrawal, suspiciousness and threats).

Young adults may present with persistent changes in functioning, behaviour or personality (withdrawal) but without marked psychotic symptoms.

Diagnostic features

The WHO Guide lists these as recent onset of:

- hallucinations (false or imagined sensations, e.g. hearing voices when no-one is around)
- delusions (firmly held ideas that are often false and not shared by others in the patient's social, cultural or ethnic group, e.g. patients may believe they are being poisoned by neighbours, receiving messages from the television or being looked at by others in some special way)
- disorganised or strange speech
- agitation or bizarre behaviour
- extreme and labile emotional states.

It is essential to listen to the family, as this will assist in the diagnosis. Before a diagnosis of schizophrenia can be made, other causes for the symptoms need to be excluded. These include drug misuse, alcoholic hallucinations, severe infections or febrile illness and epilepsy. Patients who present with the above symptoms for the first time will need urgent referral to specialist services.

The symptoms of schizophrenia are often described as:

- positive – hallucinations, delusions, thought interference, behavioural problems
- negative – poor motivation, lack of drive
- thought disorder – muddled or disconnected speech.

Aggression and irritability may be a feature of schizophrenia though serious offences are rare. Aggression is more likely in conjunction with acute disorder and may be associated with drug or alcohol misuse. Early intervention and accessible 24-hour services are important factors which reduce the likelihood of aggressive behaviour getting out of hand.[3]

There has been much debate over the years about the causes of schizophrenia, with some people expressing doubts as to whether it exists at all. More recent research is demonstrating that this and similar conditions are in fact diseases of the central nervous system and that there are changes in brain chemistry and clear abnormalities present in people with severe forms. There is also a strong genetic component. The picture is extremely complex, but previous beliefs that schizophrenia was the result purely of social and environmental influences, in particular dysfunctional families, have been shown to be very wide of the mark.[4]

Care of people with schizophrenia

This does not mean that the treatment of schizophrenia is confined to medication. Medication plays an important part but psychological and social interventions are also vital in an illness which has such devastating effects on both the individual and their families. Modern approaches to care encompass all these elements within the framework provided by the Care Programme Approach (*see* p. 80). The fact is that most people with serious mental illness are nowadays cared for within the community, and most will be registered with a GP. Primary care staff, including nurses, need to take the care of this highly vulnerable group of people very seriously.

A consensus group, convened some time before the publication of the National Service Framework, identified five areas of care in which primary care needed to be involved.[5] These remain relevant.

1   Identifying patients and organising regular review (this is a requirement under the National Service Framework).
2   Comprehensive assessments including social and environmental factors, mental state, physical problems and medication.
3   Provision of information and advice for patients and carers.
4   Clear indications for involvement of specialist services.
5   Arrangements for crisis management.

Not all primary care teams will want to do all of this. What is important is that it is done and that responsibilities are clear. The ideal arrangements will be some form of shared care between the primary care team and the CMHT. Many primary care teams will probably be most closely involved in providing physical healthcare. People with serious mental illness are just as much entitled to care for their asthma, diabetes, hypertension and arthritis as other patients. Moreover, they are also entitled to preventive interventions such as cervical cytology, nutritional advice and help with smoking cessation.

Medication

Antipsychotics are the main drug treatment for psychoses. There are a wide variety of these drugs in use, many of them older preparations ('typical antipsychotics' or 'neuroleptics') which are often unpopular with patients and may have serious side effects. Treatment adherence is a serious problem with these drugs, often due to such side effects as akathisia (severe restlessness), sedation, weight gain and sexual dysfunction.[6] Other side effects include parkinsonian-type symptoms and tardive dyskinesia. The latter is characterised by involuntary movements, usually of face and tongue, but sometimes of the whole body. Most side effects are reversible, either by stopping the antipsychotic, or by adding other drugs, e.g. anti-parkinsonian drugs. Tardive dyskinesia may be permanent. Good practice in the use of antipsychotics suggests that patients should be prescribed only one of these drugs and that it should be used in the smallest dose possible consistent with effective treatment. Drugs of this type include those commonly given as depot preparations: haloperidol (Haldol), flupenthixol (Depixol) and fluphenazine (Modecate).

More recently, more modern drugs such as risperidone, olanzapine and clozapine have appeared on the scene. Though more expensive than the older drugs they are claimed to be more effective, have fewer side effects and are more acceptable to patients. Clozapine is usually used for the treatment of resistant schizophrenia, with some success. Many newly diagnosed patients are likely to be prescribed one of these drugs.

Antipsychotics are effective in controlling positive symptoms, but may need to be taken over long periods of time in order to prevent relapse. Some people who have had a diagnosis for many years may be on depot neuroleptics. These are given by intramuscular injection, and only have to be given every few weeks. Research has confirmed that many practice nurses are giving these drugs on a regular basis, but as Gray and colleagues found in a national survey, drug side effects were rarely monitored.[7] In view of the potential seriousness of the side effects of these drugs, this finding is extremely worrying. Anecdotal evidence also suggests that a number of these patients may have no contact with any professional other than a practice nurse.

Practice nurses who have no training in this field may feel it more appropriate to question whether they are competent to give these drugs at all.

Bipolar disorder

This condition may also be known as bipolar depression or manic depression. Patients experience episodes of depression and mania, sometimes together, sometimes alternately.[8] Patients may not realise they are ill and because of this lack of insight, help may be requested by relatives or friends. The WHO Guide lists the diagnostic features as follows.

- Periods of mania with:
  - increased energy and activity
  - elevated mood or irritability
  - rapid speech
  - loss of inhibitions
  - decreased need for sleep
  - increased importance of self.

- The patient may be easily distracted.

- The patient may also have periods of depression with:
  - low or sad mood
  - loss of interest or pleasure.

- The following associated symptoms are frequently present:
  - disturbed sleep
  - guilt or low self-worth
  - fatigue or loss of energy
  - poor concentration
  - disturbed appetite
  - suicidal thoughts or acts.

Either type of episode may predominate. Episodes may alternate frequently or may be separated by periods of normal mood. Patients may have hallucinations or delusions during periods of mania or depression.

People with bipolar disorder can be difficult to treat and to help. During the manic phase they may be irresponsible with money, sexually promiscuous and reject support. Depressions may be severe and the risk of suicide may be high. In recent years it has become apparent that at least some people with this condition can learn to manage it themselves, in much the same way as a person with diabetes learns to manage their condition. Guinness suggests that people who learn self-management have less frequent and less severe mood swings, are more tolerant of stress and may have more stable relationships and better employment prospects.[9] Details of these techniques are available from the Manic Depression Fellowship (*see* Appendix).

Lithium salts are often used as a mood stabiliser in bipolar disorder. They are highly toxic and since they are used for long periods, sometimes for life, patients require three-monthly blood tests and medical examinations to ensure that blood levels are stable within a narrow range.[8] Side effects include tremor, blurred vision, excessive passing of urine, excessive thirst, anorexia, vomiting, diarrhoea, mild drowsiness or sluggishness, giddiness and poor co-ordination, slurring, eye problems, kidney problems and seizures. Most of these are reversible if the drug is reduced or temporarily stopped, but patients need to know that they should seek medical advice if the effects persist or get worse. Long-term use of the drug may be associated with changes in kidney function and thyroid and skin or heart problems.

Puerperal psychosis

This severe condition affects about 1 in 500 women following childbirth. The onset is normally rapid, usually within the first two weeks following delivery. The incidence has remained unchanged for many years and is constant in many countries. Most of the literature suggests that hospital admission is almost always required, usually mother and baby together in order to preserve the essential bonding. Mothers with the condition may be managed at home where there is close collaboration between health visitor and CPN.

The diagnosis of puerperal psychosis is confusing. The associated psychotic symptoms are not always similar to those encountered in other psychoses, but there is evidence to suggest that they may be more dramatic and severe.[10] The causes are similarly obscure and much more research is needed. Most women, for whom the episode of puerperal psychosis is the first psychotic episode, make a full recovery, but there is a risk of recurrence in future pregnancies.

Treatment may be with antipsychotic medication, as for schizophrenia, but will vary according to the symptoms shown by the individual. Electroconvulsive therapy (ECT) may be used, and may bring rapid improvement in some patients. Patients will need a great deal of support following discharge from hospital, which will involve health visitors working in close collaboration with CMHT members.

The Care Programme Approach

The Care Programme Approach (CPA) which was introduced in 1991, is a comprehensive framework for assessing the health and social needs of people who suffer mental health problems. Considerable confusion has arisen over the past few years about the implementation of the CPA and how it fits in with the parallel system of care management operated by social service departments.[11] The National Service Framework has attempted to clarify the issues. Standards 4 and 5 now state that there should be integration of care management and CPA, with two levels of CPA.

These are:

- standard CPA – this is for people who require the intervention of only one agency or discipline and who are no danger to themselves or anyone else. These are people who would not be at high risk if they lost contact with services.
- enhanced CPA – this is for people with multiple needs and who require more intensive help. These are often people with whom maintaining contact is difficult and who would be likely to pose a risk if contact was lost.

All individuals on the CPA require a written care plan, agreed with the patient and their carers, but those on enhanced CPA will have much more detailed plans. These plans should include:

- arrangements for mental healthcare including medication
- assessment of risk with contingency plans
- arrangements for physical healthcare (usually by GP)

- action needed to secure appropriate accommodation, domestic support if required, employment, education, training or other occupation
- arrangements for adequate income
- provision for cultural and faith needs
- promotion of independence and social contact including any therapeutic leisure activities
- date of next planned review.

This care plan should be drawn up by a named care co-ordinator (previously called the 'key worker'), with the involvement of the service user (patient) and their carer where appropriate. A copy should be given to the GP. It is particularly important that crisis arrangements are accessible to everyone who is likely to have contact with this person, including GP out-of-hours services and locums. Most people in this category will probably not be receiving depot neuroleptic medication from a practice nurse, but if they are, review is essential. CPA involves all services likely to come into contact with users, including the criminal justice system.

Working together: primary care and specialist services

Most of the highly publicised failures in care for severely mentally ill people have been shown by subsequent enquiries to be the result of failures in communication between professionals. In *Building Bridges* (1995) the government at the time acknowledged the important role of primary care teams in providing care for this group of patients and suggested that specialist services had an important training role with primary care teams.[12] Goldberg and Gournay also thought that this was an important part of the responsibility of specialist teams.[13] In practice, developments along these lines have been patchy for a number of reasons, including lack of training skills on the part of CMHT members, lack of understanding of the primary care setting and poor management support for the training role.

There have, however, been a number of other developments, which may involve an element of education and training, but which also focus on building links between primary care teams and community mental health teams.

The Bradford model

In Bradford, West Yorkshire, Health Action Zone funding has allowed the employment of three primary care liaison nurses, one to each primary care trust (PCT). These nurses are based in the CMHTs which are co-terminus with the PCTs.

The key roles of these posts are as follows.

- Education: delivering educational packages at practice and PCT level.
- Assisting individuals to develop skills in cognitive behaviour therapy and solution focused therapy.
- Guideline development and implementation as required by the National Service Framework.
- Improving communication between primary care teams and CMHTs. For example there has been an audit of communication, forums which include service users have been set up and there have been individual practice meetings with the CMHT.
- The development in primary care of registers for those suffering from severe and enduring mental health problems.

The nurses have also been able to examine current service provision and look at new ways of delivering primary mental health care. New clinics have been established which are staffed by non-medical personnel, usually primary care nurses, health visitors, social workers, community psychiatric nurses, and primary care service users. A GP who is trained as a mental health GP specialist is present through the clinic and provides supervision. The team have been trained in solution focused therapy and the locally agreed risk assessment method. They have developed their own assessment tool.

The clinics deal with people who have mild to moderate mental health problems that would not be severe enough for referral to secondary care, but whose problems are too complex to be dealt with in a normal GP consultation. All patients who are referred to the clinic are offered an initial assessment. The assessment is discussed at the end of the clinic with the whole team, including the GP, and a decision about further intervention is made. The clinic has links with the wider community and was timed to run at the same time as a session run by a benefits advice worker at the same health centre.

Primary care held CPA registers have been implemented so that each practice is able to identify the patients that are on the CPA. A template attached to the practice computer system has also been developed to assist with information such as the annual physical health check, the care coordinator and the action required if the care programme breaks down.

The nurses have been an essential link between primary care and the local implementation team for the National Service Framework, representing the voice of primary care.

The Woodlands two branch model

As with the Bradford model, the Woodlands CMHT have recognised that whilst it is important to prioritise those patients with severe mental illness, people with less severe illness also require help, and that these people form an important part of the primary care clientele. They have developed a system which provides support to primary care teams in the care of people with mild to moderate symptoms, but which does not compromise the care of more seriously ill patients. The CMHT has two branches, one dealing with severe mental illness, the other with assessment and short-term intervention. Each branch is separate, with different personnel.

They describe the key points of their service as:

- ensuring services address all aspects of mental healthcare delivery
- ensuring that those with the most severe needs are prioritised
- team respect for branch existence
- primary and secondary care in partnership
- streamlined use of professional skills and training
- answering and not ignoring a problem
- decision making about outcome following face-to-face contact.

They have developed a detailed referral guide for primary care which includes the option of advice to the primary care team as to whether referral is appropriate or not. Where referrals are not appropriate, they can advise on alternative sources of help for patients. They also provide educational input for primary care teams and for patients.

(Information from Elaine Walker, Team leader, Blackpool, Wyre and Fylde Community Health Services NHS Trust.)

Conclusion

These two models illustrate some of the innovative work that is happening around the country to break down the artificial barriers that have existed for too long between primary and secondary care services for people with mental health problems. Primary care nurses need to be involved in these developments and need to understand the systems that are being put in place under the National Service Framework. It is professionally unacceptable not to know the CPN who visits the practice, to be unaware of the contact arrangements for people on the CPA and not to know how to contact the local crisis team.

Standards 2 and 3 of the National Service Framework are about primary care services for people with mental health problems. Primary care organisations are designated lead agencies for the implementation of these standards. That means they should be pro-active and not wait for someone else to tell them what they should be doing. The danger of sitting back is that the services which are put in place will not meet the needs of people in primary care, patients or professionals. Primary care nurses have a vital part to play in this and need to be involved.

References

1   Strathdee G and Kendrick T (1996) Regular review of schizophrenia. In: T Kendrick, A Tylee and P Freeling (eds) *The Prevention of Mental Illness in Primary Care*. Cambridge University Press, Cambridge.

2   Kendrick T (1996) Organising continuing care of the long-term mentally ill in general practice. In: T Kendrick, A Tylee and P Freeling (eds) *The Prevention of Mental Illness in Primary Care*. Cambridge University Press, Cambridge.

3   Kingdon D (2000) Schizophrenia and mood (affective) disorder. In: D Bailey (ed.) *At the Core of Mental Health: key issues for practitioners, managers and mental health trainers*. Pavilion Publishing, Brighton.

4   Gournay K (1995) New facts on schizophrenia. *Nursing Times*. **91**(25): 32–3.

5   Burns T and Kendrick T (1997) The primary care of patients with schizophrenia: a search for good practice. *Br J Gen Pract*. **47**: 515–20.

6   Peveler R (1999) Encouraging concordance with treatment for depression and schizophrenia. *Community Ment Health*. **2**(3): 5–7.

7   Gray R, Parr A-M, Plummer S *et al.* (1999) A national survey of practice nurse involvement in mental health interventions. *J Adv Nurs.* **30**(4): 901–6.

8   Wilkinson G, Moore B and Moore P (1999) *Treating People with Depression: a practical guide for primary care.* Radcliffe Medical Press, Oxford.

9   Guinness D (1997) A guide to self-management. In: V Varma (ed.) *Managing Manic Depressive Disorders.* Jessica Kingsley Publishers, London.

10 Riley D (1995) Puerperal psychosis (Chapter 6). In: *Perinatal Mental Health: a source book for health professionals.* Radcliffe Medical Press, Oxford.

11 Bailey D (2000) Care planning and care co-ordination in mental health. In: D Bailey (ed.) *At the Core of Mental Health: key issues for practitioners, managers and mental health trainers.* Pavilion Publishers, Brighton.

12 DoH (1995) *Building Bridges: a guide to arrangements for inter-agency working for the care and protection of severely mentally ill people.* Department of Health, London.

13 Goldberg D and Gournay K (1997) *The General Practitioner, the Psychiatrist and the Burden of Mental Health Care.* Maudsley discussion paper No. 1. Institute of Psychiatry, London.

Further reading

For more information on antipsychotic drugs and their side effect profiles, *see*: *The Maudsley Prescribing Guidelines* (5e) (1999). Martin Dunitz, London.

Brooker C and Repper J (eds) (1998) *Serious Mental Health Problems in the Community.* Baillière Tindall, London.

Inside Out: a guide to self-management of manic depression. Available from the Manic Depression Fellowship, 8–10 High St, Kingston-on-Thames, Surrey KT1 1EY.

Copeland ME (1994) *Living Without Depression and Manic Depression: a workbook for maintaining mood stability.* New Harbinger Press, USA.

CHAPTER SEVEN

Mental illness in older people

Bev Hallpike

Introduction

The recently published National Service Framework for Older People sets eight standards of care including Standard 7 which is specifically about care for older people with mental health problems.[1] This standard states that older people are entitled to access to integrated mental health services to ensure effective diagnosis, treatment and support for them and their carers. In addition, Standard 1 is designed to root out age discrimination and specifically states that NHS services will be provided on the basis of clinical need alone. Standard 2, which is about person-centred care, says that the NHS and social services should treat older people as individuals and enable them to make choices about their care. This chapter will address all of these issues, with a particular focus on the contribution to be made by primary care nurses.

In recent years there has been an explosion of knowledge on the subject of dementia and depression in the lives of older people. While it must be acknowledged that other mental health problems such as anxiety, phobias, paraphrenia and confusional states still feature, depression and dementia are the most prominent. The main focus of this chapter will therefore be on issues of dementia with support for carers. It will begin by looking at ways of combating depression in later life.

Depression

Depression is the most common mental health problem in the elderly and is said to be under-diagnosed and under-treated. The clinical features of depression in the elderly are the same as in younger patients. However, presentation may differ and diagnosis may be made more difficult due to symptoms of physical illnesses or masked co-morbid anxiety or dementia. Depression is not an integral part of the ageing process. This commonly held myth has perhaps arisen because many elderly people have concurrent medical problems or somatic symptoms with no known cause and which never seem to get better. There are also a number of losses encountered in old age, which may leave the elderly with a sense of foreboding.

Patients with depression commonly complain to the doctor or nurse of physical symptoms such as pain or being tired all the time. Somatic presentations may be especially likely in older people. The diagnostic features are those listed in Chapter 1:

- low or sad mood
- loss of interest or pleasure

and four or more of the following:

- disturbed sleep pattern
- disturbed appetite
- guilt or low self-worth
- pessimism or hopelessness about the future
- decreased libido
- diurnal mood variation
- poor concentration
- suicidal thoughts or acts
- loss of self-confidence
- fatigue or loss of energy
- agitation or slowing of movement or speech.

Depression may be linked with anxiety symptoms, unexplained physical complaints and alcohol or drug misuse.[2]

Research studies have revealed that 2–4% of older people suffer from major depression with suicide being particularly common in this group. It is estimated that around 25% of suicides in the UK are people over the age of 65, with older men at particular risk.[3] About half of these people may have actually seen a health professional within the last week of their lives. The question then arises 'Why was depression missed?'.

The reasons are likely to be similar to those discussed in Chapter 1, with the addition of widespread ageist beliefs. These attitudes are not helped by the pervasive media portrayal of old age as all doom and gloom. There appears to be a general notion that depression in later life is normal or justified as a result of various losses, chronic illness, loneliness or social isolation. Pitt suggests that this assumption is a major barrier to the recognition of depression.[4]

Assessment

The key tasks in the assessment of depression in older people are essentially similar to those in younger people. It is important to check the following:

KEY TASKS

Assess: SEVERITY

                DURATION

                       SOCIAL NETWORK

                           PAST HISTORY

                               VIEWS OF SELF

                                   SUICIDAL THINKING

As for younger people, screening tools may be helpful. There are a variety of validated instruments which could be used:

- the GDS (Geriatric Depression Scale)[5]
- the HAM-D (Hamilton Depression rating scale)[6]
- the Beck Depression Inventory[7]
- the Zung Self Depression Scale.[8]

The GDS is probably the ideal screening tool for primary care settings, as it is easy to use and no psychiatric expertise is required. Designed to elicit a simple yes/no response, it can be used by doctors, nurses and any member of the CMHT. The flexibility of the GDS enables application in any setting – hospital, surgery, residential setting or in the home. The GDS evaluates clinical severity of depression and is useful in monitoring the patient during treatment. Yesavage suggests it also works well in mild to moderate dementia with its focus on the cognitive aspects of depressive illness as opposed to physical symptoms.[5] This scale may be used as part of the over-75 health check.

Box 7.1   GERIATRIC DEPRESSION SCALE (GDS)
(15-item version)

Please circle the answer which applies to you.

Are you basically satisfied with your life?	Yes/NO
Have you dropped many of your activities and interests?	YES/No
Do you feel that your life is empty?	YES/No
Do you often get bored?	YES/No
Are you in good spirits most of the time?	Yes/NO
Are you afraid that something bad is going to happen to you?	YES/No
Do you feel happy most of the time?	Yes/NO
Do you often feel helpless?	YES/No
Do you prefer to stay at home, rather than going out and doing new things?	YES/No
Do you feel you have more problems with memory than most?	YES/No
Do you think it is wonderful to be alive now?	Yes/NO
Do you feel pretty worthless the way you are now?	YES/No
Do you feel full of energy?	Yes/NO
Do you feel that your situation is hopeless?	YES/No
Do you feel that most people are better off than you are?	YES/No

Box 7.2   How to score the GDS

Each answer in capitals scores 1 point. All other answers score 0.

0–4:   not depressed
5–15:   may be suffering from a depressive illness. Requires further assessment.

From: Katona *et al.* (1995).[9]

Risk factors which should be considered include:

- personal history/family history of depression
- bereavement
- dementia (people with dementia may also suffer from depression)
- poor physical health/disability, especially sight or hearing loss, chronic pain, terminal illness
- certain medication (benzodiazepines, propanalol, cimetidine)
- loneliness
- poverty/financial worries
- being a carer of someone with a chronic illness (note recent changes in carer's health or consulting behaviour).

Treatment issues

Depression in the elderly should be treated with the same diligence as any other illness. It is important to assess both physical and mental health. Depression in the elderly is often associated with physical illness, especially chronic, disabling conditions. The condition may be secondary to physical problems such as congestive heart failure, stroke, back pain or bronchitis. Some neurological conditions, such as Parkinson's disease and some endocrine disorders such as hypothyroidism, may lead to symptoms similar to depression. Treating the physical condition may improve depressive symptoms; treating depression may improve physical symptoms.

Older people in residential homes are more likely to suffer depression than those in the community. Up to 40% of residents in care suffer hearing loss, 45% suffer visual impairment, both of which serve to reduce communication and increase isolation. Elderly residents have often suffered reduction in mobility and capability and may be incontinent, leading to feelings of dependence, helplessness, loss of dignity and self-esteem. Addressing some of these issues can have a profound effect on mental state. Treating depression is also likely to reduce unnecessary demands on primary care teams and improve the morale of carers.

For an outline of currently available antidepressant medication *see* Chapter 1. The management of depression in general practice has tremendous cost implications, especially the treatment of older people who may need to stay on medication for longer than younger people. The tricyclic antidepressants (TCAs) have been used as first line treatment for many years. They are effective and until recently were much cheaper than newer antidepressants but they may not always be appropriate for elderly people.

Special precautions may need to be taken because of the side effects profile. Elderly patients are more vulnerable to serious side effects and they may require a lower dose than younger adults. All tricyclics have a certain degree of cardiotoxicity and should be avoided by patients with any form of heart condition. Postural hypotension has been responsible for many accidents.[10] Urinary retention may be a problem for older men with prostatism. The tricyclics are also sedating and may lead to falls and an increased risk of hip fractures.

The selective serotonin re-uptake inhibitors (SSRIs) appear to have a more rapid response rate, lower side effect profile and less toxicity rendering them less dangerous in overdose than the TCAs. This may be particularly important when prescribing for an elderly person who has suicidal ideas. These drugs are also less sedating than the TCAs. Some SSRIs are now becoming available in generic form which will reduce their cost.

Psychological and social therapies

There is growing evidence that psychological treatments have been useful for patients with milder forms of depression and even those with chronic illness. This is likely to be as true for older people as it is for younger patients. Supportive psychotherapy is often undervalued, as its efficacy is not easily measurable. Lovestone and Howard believe that cognitive behavioural therapy is likely to be a particularly appropriate form of therapy for older people with its focus on correcting dysfunctional forms of thinking.[11] Cognitive behavioural therapy has proven to be effective, particularly in phobias and depressive anxiety states and shows reduction in hospital readmission rates as a result of group therapy. A combination of cognitive behavioural therapy and medication may be particularly useful.[12] Focused bereavement counselling also has its place.

Patients often indicate their preference for 'counselling' rather than drug treatment. Anecdotal evidence suggests they value a set time when they are listened to and given positive encouragement. Many of the techniques outlined in Chapter 3 will be helpful with elderly people. There are suggestions that group methods may be especially useful, but that older people may do best in therapeutic groups which cater specifically for their needs, rather than in mixed age groups.

Social interventions, such as encouraging engagement in self-help or support groups, attendance at structured day activities (e.g. local clubs, Age Concern centres), art clubs, creative writing classes or regular sessions at a local leisure centre, all help to combat isolation and loneliness and build self-esteem and confidence.

Dementia

Dementia is a term that describes a group of varying brain disorders that result in the progression of severe memory loss. The World Health Organization (WHO) defines dementia as the global impairment of higher cortical functions, including memory, the capacity to solve problems of day-to-day living, the performance of learned perception, motor skills, the correct use of social skills and control of emotional reactions, in the absence of gross 'clouding of consciousness'. The condition is often irreversible and progressive.[13]

There are various types of dementia:

- Alzheimer's disease
- vascular dementia
- Lewy body dementia
- fronto-temporal dementia
- subcortical dementias (i.e. Parkinson's disease or Huntingdon's chorea)
- Creutzfeld Jakob disease
- neuro-AIDS
- alcohol-related dementia
- genetic abnormality, e.g. Down's syndrome.

Alzheimer's disease is the most common cause of dementia, accounting for 50–60% of cases.[14] No two persons are affected in the same way. The impact of the illness may be manifested according to the person's premorbid personality traits. The prevalence of dementia appears to be higher in females than males particularly from the age of 75 onwards.[15] Recent estimations imply one in two people over the age of 85 will probably develop dementia.

Diseases of the cardiovascular system are important risk factors. Dementia may follow a stroke. Transient ischaemic attacks (TIAs) are often a problem particularly for those suffering heart disease, ischaemic and haemorrhagic brain lesions. Vascular dementia (multi-infarct) represents 20% of cases and is the second most common cause.[16]

During the past decade more attention has been paid to the inclusion of Lewy bodies (senile plaques) in the cortical neurones of dementia sufferers. The main clinical features of this condition are a progressive cognitive deterioration and visual hallucinations whilst Alzheimer's-type changes are absent. In addition, there are often Parkinsonian features present. Syncopal attacks and delusions may occur.

Other causes

Correct diagnosis in the elderly can often be extremely difficult but there are some treatable causes which amount to approximately 10% of those with a provisional diagnosis of dementia.[17]

Some of these include:

- depression – pseudo-dementia
- hypothyroidism
- vitamin B6 deficiency
- vitamin B12 deficiency
- acute confusional state (*see* p. 98).

Assessment

Primary care practitioners are at the front line in meeting elderly people with dementia and their carers. Dementia sufferers may remain undiagnosed until a late stage. A crisis may occur such as an illness or a bereavement which exacerbates the features and not only brings distress but reveals the inability of the sufferer or carer to cope. The essentials of good practice and robust management of dementia in the community are early detection, diagnosis and treatment as appropriate.

A coordinated and systematic assessment conducted and applied with sensitivity should provide a foundation for individually tailored care, reducing stress and the burden of care for the family and carers. It is important to obtain a good history from a reliable source. It may be important to compare the perceptions of the patient and the carer.

The following are a variety of assessment tools which may help.

- Mini-Mental State Examination (MMSE)[18]
- Alzheimer's Disease Assessment Scale (ADAS) – cognitive and non-cognitive sections (ADAS Cog, ADAS Non-cog)[19]
- Clock Drawing Test[20]
- Clifton Assessment Procedures for the Elderly (CAPE)[21]
- Brief Cognitive Rating Scale (BCRS)[22]
- Blessed Dementia Scale[23]
- Global Assessment of Psychiatric Symptoms (GAPS)
- Checklist Differentiating Pseudodementia from Dementia[24]
- Hamilton Depression Rating Scale (HAM-D)[6]
- Geriatric Depression Scale (GDS).[5]

Some of the tests above can be modified rendering them more user-friendly. Primary care nurses may require special training to use some of the scales correctly. Liaison with a local specialist CPN or CMHT for older people may be helpful.

Managing dementia on the front line

Effective management is dependent on the stage of the illness. Older people with mild dementia are generally able to manage their daily lives effectively in the community with perhaps minimal support. Those suffering severe dementia may require a maximum care package or institutional care if living alone.

Criteria for effective dementia management in the community are as follows.

- Recognition of individuals with dementia and verification of early diagnosis with possible likely causes.
- Detection of treatable and reversible causes, which may imitate features of dementia.
- Over-75 health checks can offer routine screening for dementia, though screening for depression is perhaps more useful. Carers may be at risk of developing depression, and people with dementia may also become depressed.

- Provision of relevant information to patient and carer on practical management issues at home, financial entitlements and local services to improve patients' and carers' quality of life and choices. Local social services or care management teams can advise on the appropriate benefits and allowances available to patients and carers as well as coordinate home care and support including community occupational therapy for special adaptations, home assessment and safety issues such as driving.
- Offer of specialist assessment and management of the condition. Advice on the most appropriate drug treatment and monitoring provided.
- Access to specialist services, particularly in assessment and management of behavioural difficulties, the need for ongoing medical and psychiatric treatment and CPN support. As people with dementia have complex needs for both health and social care the CMHT can provide a flexible range of services to the patient and carer.
- Early treatment – start anticholinesterase inhibitors in accordance with local guidelines (generally specialist initiation). The National Institute for Clinical Excellence (NICE) guidelines suggests no initiation if the MMSE score is less than 12.[25] They also provide a guide for discontinuation.
- Provision of a contact for adequate social care needs on a 24-hour basis.
- Offer of crisis assistance for individuals suffering an acute episode of illness and immediate support for the carer.
- Referral to local Alzheimer's Society support groups. Such groups offer information on benefit entitlement and allowances, legal issues, e.g. power of attorney. Advocates can provide assistance through the benefit maze and give help in selecting respite or long-term care away from home.

Primary care staff should expect and ask for regular feedback from others involved. Having a GP link-person would serve to increase understanding of roles, improve communication and enhance the quality and effectiveness of service provision.

Primary care teams might also like to consider the following.

- Use of protected learning time to learn more about mental health issues, tools of assessment and management in the community.
- Promote use of video training package for GPs on dementia (available from the Alzheimer's Disease International).

- Establish a carers' register within the practice. Carers are entitled to an assessment of their own needs.
- Take advantage of national recognition days using health promotion, e.g. provide display boards and literature on World Mental Health Day, Alzheimer's Awareness Day, etc.
- Create a mental health pack with patient information leaflets, literature of local resources, cassettes and contact numbers.
- Display posters and have easy access to leaflets.

Depression or dementia

Depressive pseudo-dementia is a term often used to describe the patient with depression who appears to suffer memory loss. It is very difficult to differentiate the symptoms of depressive pseudo-dementia from dementia with depressive symptoms, as there is a close similarity of some symptoms (e.g. loss of short-term memory, changes in mood/personality, loss of function and loss of concentration). Table 7.1 illustrates the main differences.

Table 7.1   How to distinguish depression from dementia

Depression	*Dementia*
Abrupt onset	Insidious onset
Short duration	Long duration
Often previous psychiatric history	May have no psychiatric history
Complains of memory loss	Often unaware of memory loss
'Don't know' answers	'Near miss' answers
Diurnal mood variation, but consistent day to day	Mood fluctuations day by day
Fluctuating cognitive loss	Stable cognitive loss
May not try hard, but distressed by losses	Tries hard to perform but unconcerned
Memory loss equal for recent and remote events	Memory loss worse for recent events
Depressed mood occurs first	Memory loss occurs first
Associated with anxiety, sleep disturbance, appetite disturbance and suicidal thoughts	May be unsociable, uncooperative, hostile, emotionally unstable, confused and disoriented. Alertness reduced

Adapted from Ham (1997).[26]

Even if diagnosis is not conclusive, the depressive symptoms should be treated, preferably with an SNRI or SSRI antidepressant.

Other conditions

Schizophrenia

Schizophrenia is a severe disorder characterised by a disintegration of thought processes, loss of contact with reality and diminished emotional responsiveness (*see* Chapter 6). It is suggested that 1–2% of older people may suffer from paranoid schizophrenic symptoms. These include people who have grown old with the illness and others who become ill later in life. People affected tend to be female, often independent and difficult to engage in health or social services. However, some older sufferers may have spent many years in hospital. Following the closure of large institutions, they may be living in supported lodgings or small group homes.

Elderly psychotic patients should receive the same standard of treatment, care and support as their younger counterparts. Compliance with treatment, and side effects of drugs, particularly extra-pyramidal effects should be monitored to prevent relapse. Many patients with psychosis experience a prodromal syndrome of identifiable symptoms as they relapse. This is known as the patient's 'relapse signature'. Early intervention in the prodrome can prevent further relapse. In some areas older patients with psychosis will be receiving depot neuroleptic medication from a practice nurse. This is an ideal opportunity to monitor a vulnerable group who are at risk of developing tardive dyskinesia.[27] It is useful, and a mark of best practice, for the primary care team to keep a record of the patient's relapse signature and a list of contact numbers as a relapse prevention strategy.

Confusional states

Confusion is not a disease but a side effect of other problems. It would appear heartless and negligent to see a young person suddenly behaving out of character, demonstrating intellectual deterioration or putting themselves or others at risk, and not seek to help or take corrective action. Yet

when this happens with an older person it is often regarded as acceptable –
'Well, what do you expect at his age?'.

Confusion can be classified into two categories:

- acute: of relatively recent onset (usually rapid)
- chronic: relatively slow onset as in a dementing illness, occurring over
  several years.

Acute confusion has three main causes:

- Physical disease – infection, often chest or urinary tract; coronary
  heart disease; multi-infarcts (minor strokes); sensory impairment
  such as hearing deficits or poor vision; carcinoma; hypothermia; re-
  absorption of toxins due to constipation. Very often these physical
  causes are treatable but they may be overlooked.
- Drugs – some types of medication can precipitate unexpected side
  effects in older people, especially if the person had inadvertently taken
  the wrong amount, for example antipsychotics, beta-blockers, digoxin,
  tranquillisers, sedatives, steroids and alcohol. Other problems may be
  caused by taking out of date medication, polypharmacy or mixing prescribed drugs with over-the-counter preparations.
- Changes in the immediate environment – when an elderly person
  leaves their familiar surroundings to go into a residential home, hospital or respite care even for a short period confusion can occur. Psychological disturbance such as a burglary, house fire, fall or the sudden
  death of a loved one may easily precipitate a confusional episode.

Most of the above can be rectified by simple interventions and timely
advice.

The insidious onset of chronic confusion is usually of an organic nature
affecting the structure and function of the brain. A dementing illness is
the usual cause, the most common being multi-infarct dementia and Alzheimer's disease.

Caring for the carers

The government has acknowledged that carers play a key role in looking
after people with mental health problems residing in the community. With

nearly six million carers in Britain and figures rising as new cases are revealed, research indicates carers of dementia sufferers experience greater levels of stress than other carers. Many family carers do not identify themselves as 'carers' but see their role as part and parcel of their duty.

The National Service Framework for Mental Health, in Standard 6 'Caring about Carers', stipulates that apart from having their own needs assessed, carers should receive easily understandable information about both the help available to them and the services provided for the person they care for. It calls for local services to pay greater attention to the needs of carers. As primary care organisations become increasingly involved in commissioning health services, steps need to be taken to include carers. Studies indicate that carers' perceptions of services have been that they are not always appropriate. Relationships with the professionals involved are often tinged with ambiguity.[28] Carers often felt that their needs were not being addressed.

Other studies have identified certain categories of need:[29,30]

- information and support
- emotional support
- skills training
- respite care.

Effective implementation of the criteria above would ensure that most of these needs were met. Carers are entitled to a separate assessment of their own needs. Joint working with other professionals, for example district nurses and CPNs can be advantageous for all concerned, reducing the mystique of professional roles and enhancing practical skills in an opportunistic way. Carers also need to know who to contact in the time of crisis. Providing appropriate information and education can significantly reduce carer stress and increase their understanding and self-confidence in care giving.[31,32]

Elder abuse

The Department of Health described abuse of older people in domestic settings as:[33]

'Physical, sexual, psychological or financial. It may be intentional or unintentional as a result of neglect. It causes harm to the older person either temporarily or over a period of time.'

Older people with mental health problems who live alone are more vulnerable to exploitation by carers or relatives.[34] Caring for a challenging and dependent older person can be emotionally taxing and physically exhausting for the carer. If the carer has other responsibilities and commitments such as a job, spouse or children, the stresses and added pressure of caring for an elderly relative can be overwhelming. There is an increased tendency for abuse to occur in families where there have previously been abusive relationships. It is also worthy of note that even where the elderly persons are quite frail, they can also be the perpetrators of abuse.[35]

If abuse is suspected, primary care nurses need to work closely with other professionals, recording incidents of abuse and clarifying roles and responsibilities. Social service departments usually have a policy and procedure in place for elder abuse. A care manager should be able to help. In sheltered housing schemes, wardens usually have access to housing department policies and will be familiar with the issues and procedures.

Conclusion

Carers need to feel valued and better equipped if they are to continue caring. It is as well to remember that many of those caring for elderly people with dementia are spouses and therefore elderly themselves. Caring professionals have a duty to educate the public and, where necessary, develop a therapeutic alliance to ensure that the elderly receive the quality of care and dignity they deserve.

References

1 Department of Health (2001) *National Service Framework for Older People.* Department of Health, London.

2 WHO (2000) *WHO Guide to Mental Health in Primary Care* (UK Version). Royal Society of Medicine, London. www.whoguidemhpcuk.org.

3 Katona CL (1994) *Depression in Old Age.* John Wiley and Sons, Chichester.

4 Pitt B (1995) Defeating depression in old age. Cited in: C Holmes and R Howard (eds) (1997) *Advances in Old Age Psychiatry: chromosomes to community care.* Wrightson Biomedical Publishing, Petersfield.

5 Yesavage JA, Brink IL, Lum O *et al.* (1983) Development and validation of a geriatric depression screening scale. A preliminary report. *J Psychiatr Res.* 1737–49.

6 Hamilton M (1960) A rating scale for depression. *J Neurol Neurosurg Psychiatry.* **23**: 56–62.

7 Beck AT, Ward CH, Mendelson M *et al.* (1961) An inventory for measuring depression. *Arch Gen Psychiatry.* **4**: 53–63.

8 Zung WWK (1965) A self-rating depression scale. *Arch Gen Psychiatry.* **12**: 63–70.

9 Katona C, Freeling P, Blanchard M *et al.* (1995) Recognition and management of depression in late life: consensus statement. *Primary Care Psychiatry.* **1**: 107–13.

10 Ray WA (1992) Psychotropic drugs and injuries among the elderly: a review. *J Psychopharm.* **12**: 386–96.

11 Lovestone S and Howard R (1996) *Depression in Elderly People.* Martin Dunitz, London.

12 Blackburn IM, Eunson KM and Bishop S (1986) A two year naturalistic follow-up of depressed patients treated with cognitive therapy, pharmacotherapy and combination of both. *J Affect Disord.* **10**: 67–75.

13 WHO (1986) *Dementia in Later Life: research and action.* Report of a WHO scientific group on senile dementia. WHO Technical Report Series 730. World Health Organization, Geneva.

14 Henderson A (1994) *Dementia.* World Health Organization, Geneva.

15 Audit Commission (2000) *National Report: Forget Me Not.* Audit Commission, London.

16 Jorm A, Korten A and Henderson A (1987) The prevalence of dementia: a quantitative integration of the literature. *Acta Psychiatr Scand.* **76**: 465–79.

17 Alzheimer's Society (1995) *Dementia in the Community: management strategies for general practice.* Alzheimer's Society, London.

18 Folstein MF, Folstein SE and McHugh PR (1975) 'Mini-mental State': a practical method for grading the cognitive state of patients for the clinician. *J Psychiatr Res.* **12**: 189–98.

19 Rosen WG, Mohs RC and Davis KL (1984) A new rating scale for Alzheimer's disease. *Am J Psychiatry.* **141**: 1356–64.

20 Brodaty H and Moore CM (1997) The Clock Drawing Test for dementia of the Alzheimer's type: a comparison of three scoring methods in a memory disorders clinic. *Int J Geriatr Psychiatry*. **12**: 619–27.

21 Pattie AH and Gilleard CJ (1997) *Manual of the Clifton Assessment Procedures for the Elderly*. Hodder and Stoughton Education, Sevenoaks.

22 Reisberg B and Ferris SH (1988) Brief Cognitive Rating Scale. *Psychopharma Bull*. **24**: 629–36.

23 Blessed G, Tomlinson BE and Roth M (1968) The association between quantitative measures of dementia and of senile changes in the cerebral grey matter of elderly subjects. *Br J Psychol*. **114**: 797–811.

24 Wells CE (1979) Pseudodementia. *Am J Psychol*. **136**: 895–900.

25 National Institute for Clinical Excellence (2001) NICE review for cholinesterase inhibitors. Cited in: M Naidoo and R Bullock (2001) *An Integrated Care Pathway for Dementia. Best Practice for Dementia Care*.

26 Ham RJ (1997) Confusion, dementia and delirium. In: RJ Ham and PD Sloane (eds) *Primary Care Geriatrics. A case based approach* (3e). Mosby, St Louis, pp. 217–59.

27 Jeste DV, Larco JP, Gilbert PL *et al.* (1993) Treatment of late-life schizophrenia with neuroleptics. *Schizophr Bull*. **19**: 817–30.

28 Department of Health (1991) *Carer Support in the Community: evaluation of the Department of Health initiative, 'Demonstration Districts for Informal Carers' 1986–1989*. Department of Health, London.

29 Twigg J and Atkin K (1994) *Carers Perceived: policy and practice in informal care*. Open University Press, Buckingham.

30 Mudge K and Radcliffe I (1995) Considering the needs of carers: a survey of their views on services. *Nursing Standard*. **9**(30): 29–31.

31 Brodaty H and Gresham M (1989) Effects of a training programme to reduce stress in carers of patients with dementia. *BMJ*. **299**: 1375–9.

32 Jansson W, Almber B, Grafstrom M *et al.* (1998) The Circle Model: support for relatives of people with dementia. *Int J Geriatr Psychiatry*. **13**(10): 674–81.

33 Department of Health (1993) *No Longer Afraid. Abuse of Older People in Domestic Settings*. HMSO, London.

34 McCreadie C and Tinker A (1993) Review: abuse of elderly people in the domestic setting: a UK perspective. *Age Ageing*. **22**: 65–9.

35 Salomon MJ (1998) Parents who continue to abuse. *Clin Gerontol*. **18**(3): 60–3.

Further reading

Coope B, Ballard C and Saad K (1995) The prevalence of depression in the carers of dementia sufferers. *Br J Psychol.* **10**: 237–42.

Dementia in the Community: management strategies for general practice. Alzheimer's Society, Gordon House, 10 Greencoat Place, London SW1P 1PH.

Department of Health (1999) *Our Healthier Nation – Mental Health National Service Framework: Executive summary.* Department of Health, London.

Jones G and Miesen BML (1993) *Care-Giving in Dementia* (Vol 1). Routledge, London.

Norman IJ and Redfern SJ (1997) *Mental Health Care for Elderly People.* Churchill Livingstone, Edinburgh.

CHAPTER EIGHT

Stigma: discrimination, ethnicity and gender issues in primary care

Ann Mitchell

Introduction

The concept of stigma has been in existence since the creation of human kind and still prevails today in our modern society. Whitehead writes that the 'notion of stigma has always been an intrinsic part of our societies and civilisations. In modern times, the Victorian era is particularly associated with social stigma'.[1] Although some stigmas around certain diseases and disorders, for example smallpox and plague, may have been eradicated, they have been replaced by more modern stigmatising conditions such as HIV/AIDS and cancer.

Tuberculosis was once portrayed as a stigmatising condition. Society thought it had disappeared forever. However, there has been a resurgence of this disease and negative attitudes to it have once more reared their heads. A recent series of cases in a local city college received a great deal of media attention fuelling fears of a major epidemic. This sparked off a range of anxieties for children and their families, particularly those attending the college, and nearby residents. The whole notion of stigma and its negative connotations remains endemic in our society.

What is stigma?

To aid our understanding of this complex term, Goffman refers to it as an 'attribution that makes an individual appear to be different from others and it can be deeply discrediting' for the individual.[2] Goffman describes three different types of stigma in his classic text.

1   'Abominations of the body which relate to various physical deformities.' The stigma is conferred on that individual who is perceived by others as having an unattractive appearance.
2   The second stigma relates to the 'blemishes of individual character which leads to them being perceived as weak with domineering or unnatural passions. Mental disorders, imprisonment, addiction, alcoholism, suicidal attempts and radical political behaviour all fall within this category.'
3   'Tribal stigma is associated with race, nation and religion. This stigma can be transmitted through lineages and equally contaminate all members of a family.'

The assumption, based on Goffman's work, is that a person who is stigmatised is not quite human. As a consequence we use various means to discredit, discriminate against and stereotype the individual, often unthinkingly reducing their life chances.

Discrimination

The word is inextricably linked with stigma but its more defined meaning is associated with prejudging another who may appear to be different. That difference could be in terms of colour, race, mental illness or even gender. Campbell and Heginbotham suggest that 'to discriminate is to treat someone badly simply because of his or her membership of a mistakenly devalued group'.[3] Many individuals are discriminated against because they are put into these groups, not of their own volition but because society has placed them there. Discrimination is a form of social prejudice which can be immediately obvious or apparent in more subtle inherited attitudes. The individual who is discriminated against feels further disadvantaged and fails to achieve their full potential in any given society. A cycle of deprivation is set up in which low status and poverty are compounded by relentless lack of access to the opportunities enjoyed by the majority.

The link between mental illness and discrimination is well documented. It is the lack of respect from the public which causes the feelings of hopelessness and worthlessness. These in turn render the individual powerless and inadequate.

The stigma of mental illness

Mental illness is a broad term used for a range of psychiatric problems affecting individuals. These can vary from the common illnesses such as depression and anxiety disorders to the often more severe conditions of schizophrenia and manic depressive psychosis. While society has never fully accepted that people may have these conditions, the stigma and discrimination associated with them can seriously impair the quality of their lives. As Kaminski and Harty have highlighted, the general public sees no harm in labelling people with mental health problems as different.[4] This view will distort sufferers' self-perception, undermine their confidence and influence the way in which others relate to them.

Many people find it difficult to imagine what it must be like to be mentally ill in our affluent society. Even when they experience such an illness themselves, many people keep it a secret from their family, friends and even their GP. If and when they do disclose their problems, they may call it a 'nervous breakdown' or just 'nerves'. The fear of being labelled not quite 'normal' prevents them from revealing it more widely. Mental illness is still shrouded in secrecy, fear and ignorance. Much work needs to be done in raising awareness in a more positive way.

Stigma associated with mental illness not only affects and discriminates against members of the host community, it equally affects the minority groups living in this country.

Stigma of race

Britain has been, is, and will continue to be, a multiracial society with individuals from a range of ethnic backgrounds with differing cultural needs. It has also been widely recognised and documented that these minority groups can face a number of challenges when they attempt to settle in this country. As a result, the risk of developing mental, emotional and physical health difficulties is significantly increased.[5] These groups can also be stigmatised as a result of their race, colour or ethnic background and experience the negative behaviours shown by some of the majority population. There is also evidence to suggest that ethnic minority groups meet with double discrimination when faced with mental health problems.[6] Many can be subjected to fierce hostility and rejection as a result of racist attitudes by the majority of the host country.[7]

Many members of ethnic minority groups would prefer to see culture-specific health services that may be less discriminating and more accepting of their culture-bound behaviours. However, they are aware that they may have to access mainstream services. Gauntlett and colleagues argue that 'mainstream services fail to provide appropriate care for minority groups due to cultural gaps that are missing'.[8] What is required is 'the development and delivery of a culturally appropriate service which is not an option'. It is something that should be provided to meet the specific needs of minority ethnic groups.

Specific needs of ethnic minority clients with mental health problems

Primary care professionals are the first point of contact for the general public who may be seeking help for a particular health-related problem, regardless of their colour, creed or ethnic group. With the emergence of primary care groups and more recently, primary care trusts, it will be their ultimate responsibility to provide effective care and treatment for all within their catchment area. The primary care team will be expected to fulfil the standards laid down in the National Service Framework for Mental Health, in this instance particularly Standard 1, to 'promote mental health and reduce discrimination'.

Yet it has been recognised that primary care professionals may not necessarily have the skills, knowledge and expertise to be responsive to the mental health needs of ethnic minority groups within their communities. Therefore the needs go unmet resulting in differences in expectations and treatments in the primary care setting. These differences may occur because the individual's interpretation of their mental health problem may be entirely different to that of the primary care practitioner. Culture plays a part here in defining an individual's mental illness and is the reason why it is open to misinterpretation.

Doku gives a good example of the role of culture in referring to West African societies.[9] He states that 'West African societies believe that mental and physical illness and bad luck are caused by people who have colluded with evil forces'. He questions how many practitioners would have the knowledge of this belief and explains why they consistently fail to take into account the cultural beliefs that ethnic minority groups may have.

Moreover, ethnic minorities are not just one homogeneous group. Instead, each discrete grouping has its own beliefs and value systems about what causes mental illness. Cognisance of these factors is essential. As previously discussed, many primary care practitioners may have received limited training in this area and could bring their own prejudices and ethnocentric ways of working to therapeutic situations. Doku argues that it is the western ethnocentric training which GPs, psychiatrists and other NHS professionals receive which is at the root of the problems. What, therefore, can be done to assist the primary care team to provide an improved service for their clientele from ethnic minority groups?

There are some possible strategies which could address the deficiencies.

- Recognition and acceptance of minority groups in our society: their needs are different from, but equal to, the needs of the indigenous population.
- Recognition of individuals who are subjected to particular stresses in settling in a different country (for example, refugees). This, coupled with isolation and loneliness, can lead to stress and other mental health problems.
- Raising awareness of, and confronting attitudes to, other cultures, for example the belief that western health standards are superior to those of minority ethnic groups.
- Interpreters' system in place which has representation from each minority group in the locality.

In addition, there is a need for practitioners to acquire more specific cultural skills. This might involve the ability to make a cultural assessment. Damle suggests the following factors need to be assessed:[10]

- culture life patterns
- culture values, norms and expectations
- cultural taboos and myths
- life-caring rituals and rites of passage
- folk and professional health/illness systems.

Professionals should be aware of all these things for all groups for whom they provide a service. To build further on these assessment skills, Bhui and Oladije suggest the following criteria for improving practice.[11]

- Pay attention to patients' names, how to pronounce and spell them correctly. Understand different naming systems. Offence may be taken if patients feel they are not seen as individuals.
- Do not stereotype.
- Try to understand the individual in the context of his/her personal experiences, family, social circumstances and culture.
- Have accessible and clearly presented information available in several languages, as appropriate.
- Listen to patients' views.
- Develop awareness of own feelings towards all cultures and groups.
- Do not devalue beliefs and rituals simply because you do not understand them.
- Refer to interpreters where necessary and avoid using children to speak on behalf of their parents, particularly in emotional situations.
- Recognise that there is great cultural, religious and linguistic diversity within black and ethnic minority groups. Do not treat everyone the same.
- Acknowledge the importance of the family and extended families' attitudes and value systems.

We have addressed the mental health needs of ethnic minority groups and the range of skills, knowledge and expertise that practitioners in primary care need to adopt in order to provide culturally sensitive care. Finally, we turn to issues of stigma and gender.

Stigma and gender

Women may be stigmatised within our society simply because they are women. They may experience similar negative feelings common to other disadvantaged groups. It is well documented that many women feel oppressed, marginalised and inferior in their everyday lives. These feelings are further compounded when they suffer mental health problems. It is not suggested that men do not suffer mental health problems but there is an over-representation of women in mental health services.[12]

Research has shown that more women than men are diagnosed as mentally ill or are experiencing emotional problems which affect their ability to live happy and fulfilled lives.[13] The majority of informal carers are women. Goldberg and Huxley have demonstrated that more women than men are diagnosed by GPs as suffering from psychological problems.[14] It is fair to say that when they do become ill most women access mainstream services, but many feel prejudiced within the current framework of care and would prefer to see services which are more sensitive to their gender-specific needs.

Ethnic minority women are doubly disadvantaged. Not only do they face stigma but also discrimination. Wright illustrates their plight as brought on by a number of factors such as language difficulties, inappropriate housing and community facilities and, for some, even racist attacks.[7] There is a paucity of research relating to the healthcare of ethnic minority women. There is even less on mental health issues for ethnic minority women in primary care. The National Service Framework (Standard 1) highlights the raised suicide rate amongst young Asian women and suggests that services should be planned in partnership with local communities. This principle is as important for primary care as it is for specialist mental health services.

A recent study by Schreiber and colleagues focused on the ways in which black West Indian Canadian women manage depression.[5] These authors admit that there is limited available research to assist nurses and other care providers in knowing how to meet the needs of depressed women from cultural backgrounds other than the dominant one. However, their own findings may be relevant for some minority women in British society. 'Being strong' was a common feature of the findings. By 'strong' the women meant being able to cope by finding alternative strategies. The cultural stigma of depression was significant amongst West Indians and was perceived as being worse than that within the dominant eurocentric cultural context. They admitted being afraid of going for psychiatric help because they feared they would suffer social isolation and sanctions.

In order to help women generally, Barnes and Maple suggest that health-care professionals should provide a gender sensitive service for them.[13] In primary care terms, their criteria might be adapted as follows:

- the service should take into account women's caring responsibilities for children and other dependants
- women need space and time to talk through feelings in a non-threatening environment
- supportive groups of women with similar experiences can be helpful
- provide access to sources of practical help as well as counselling, therapy and drug treatments
- ensure access to female practitioners.

Some of these ideas pose challenges for traditional ways of working in primary care. Some health centres provide play areas for children, but women often have to take their children with them when they go into the consulting or treatment room. This may provide unwelcome distractions or mean that difficult issues may not be mentioned. The health needs of women caring for spouses, parents or disabled relatives may not be met if they are unable to leave the person they care for in order to attend the GP surgery.

Time is a major problem for GPs and nurses in primary care, but the pressure always to reduce the time available for consultations may be counterproductive. Some nurses in primary care are developing new methods of providing care for people with mental health problems which allow more time for assessment and follow-up. Health visitors have traditionally made good use of groups to provide support for mothers. There is clearly scope for other sorts of support groups within primary care, including closer collaboration with voluntary groups within the community. These groups can often provide practical help but alternatives may be access to the Citizens Advice Bureau or benefits advisers within health centres.

Most GP practices and health centres have female partners these days and women are usually free to request a female GP if they wish. There may be difficulties for some single-handed practices where the doctor is male. In some instances, they may employ a female practice nurse or nurse practitioner, but this issue may need to be addressed more creatively by primary care groups in areas with large numbers of single-handed male doctors.

Conclusion

Thus there are many issues facing primary care practitioners in seeking to provide equitable and non-stigmatising care for an often very diverse client group. Whilst nurses and others may know about many of the issues raised in this chapter, they will need to be aware of, and avoid the temptation to be influenced by, peer groups and long held prejudices. Whitehead provides some practical hints for improving practice:[1]

- work from a holistic framework of care
- consider the way stigma affects personality
- provide accessible information for patients and the general public to lessen fears and ignorance

- learn about health and sickness in other cultures
- develop interpersonal skills particularly in self-awareness and sensitivity
- set up a team forum to examine own attitudes and beliefs and those of the whole team, including reception staff.

A simple way to remember the sequence and key points of dealing with stigmatisation is to remember the following mnemonic.

- **S**elf-awareness: the skill of self-awareness lies in the individual recognising their limitations in caring for ethnic minority individuals. Primary care staff can take steps to seek appropriate courses and workshops which will equip them with the necessary knowledge, skills and sensitivity.
- **T**reatment: it is important to ensure that the prescribed treatment is tailored to meet individual needs. A sensitive approach is necessary to promote compliance.
- **I**ntuition: do not act on impulse but take adequate time to gather evidence about the individual. Ensure that you go through the appropriate channels to obtain relevant and impartial information.
- **G**ender: be aware of gender issues amongst ethnic minority women. For example, Moslem women prefer to be seen by female practitioners, not male.
- **M**ulti-cultural: primary care staff need opportunities to develop awareness of the mental health needs of the different ethnic groups living in our society, especially those living locally.
- **A**ssessment: a holistic and sensitive assessment is particularly important when dealing with mental health issues. Primary care staff need to be aware of questions which may be perceived as threatening or inappropriate. When you do not share a common language with your patient, do ensure that you have access to a professional interpreter.

References

1   Whitehead E (1995) Prejudice in practice. *Nursing Times.* **91**(21): 40–1.

2   Goffman E (1963) *Stigma.* Penguin Books, Middlesex.

3   Campbell T and Heginbotham C (1991) *Mental Illness, Prejudice, Discrimination and the Law.* Dartmouth Publishing Company Ltd, Aldershot.

4 Kaminski P and Harty C (1999) From stigma to strategy. *Nursing Standard.* **13**(38): 36–40.

5 Schrieber R, Stern PN and Charmaine W (1998) The contexts for managing depression and its stigma among black West Indian Canadian women. *J Adv Nurs.* **27**: 510–17.

6 Fernando S (1991) *Mental Health, Race and Culture.* Macmillan, London.

7 Wright J (1991) Counselling at the cultural interface: is getting back to roots enough? *J Adv Nurs.* **16**: 92–100.

8 Gauntlett N, Ford R, Johnson N *et al.* (1995) Meeting the mental heath needs of ethnic minority groups. *Nursing Times.* **91**(42): 36–7.

9 Doku J (1990) Approach to cultural awareness. *Nursing Times.* **86**(39): 69–70.

10 Damle A (undated) *Transcultural Issues in Community Psychiatry.* Unpublished.

11 Bhui K and Oladije D (1999) *Mental Health Service Provision for a Multi-cultural Society.* WB Saunders, London.

12 Prior M (1999) *Gender and Mental Health.* Macmillan, London.

13 Barnes M and Maple N (1992) *Women and Mental Health.* Venture Press, Birmingham.

14 Goldberg D and Huxley P (1980) *Mental Illness in the Community: the pathway to psychiatric care.* Tavistock, London.

Further reading

Fernando S (1991) *Mental Health, Race and Culture.* Macmillan, London.

Bugra D and Bahl V (1999) *Ethnicity: an agenda for mental health.* Gaskell, London.

Henley A and Schott J (1999) *Culture, Religion, Patient Care in a Multi-ethnic Society.* Age Concern, London.

CHAPTER NINE

Developing a team strategy

Elizabeth Armstrong

Introduction

The care of people with mental health problems in primary care has been very much a hit and miss affair over the years. It has been largely dependent on the interest and concern of individual members of primary care teams. It remains the case that if the GPs in a practice are not interested in mental health and do not believe that mental health care is part of their role, other members of the team are likely to find it very difficult to provide appropriate care.

The National Service Framework for Mental Health, which gives specific responsibilities to primary care organisations and teams, should gradually change the situation. Eventually, people with mental health problems will be able to expect that, wherever they go for help, the help they receive will meet their needs in accordance with the guiding principles set out in the framework. But the implementation of the framework is intended to be a ten-year programme. Meanwhile, the nature of primary care is changing and it will not stand still until the targets are met.

In ten years' time, primary healthcare may look very different from the system we have now. In fact primary care is not really a system at all, but a series of varying organisations providing health or medical care which have largely developed for historical reasons. Though in many areas single-handed medical practice has given way to group practices and health centres, GPs remain independent contractors to the NHS, not salaried employees. General medical practice was, and is, a business. This has nothing to do with the advent of fundholding, which is now defunct. Thus the culture of a large part of primary care is very different from the culture of the rest of the NHS.

Community nurses, such as district nurses and health visitors, have been 'attached' to designated GP practices in most areas for many years, though normally keeping their own, separate management structure. Being employed directly by NHS organisations, these nurses have often enjoyed better conditions of service than their practice nurse colleagues. Practice nurses have historically been directly employed by GPs. This fragmentation of the nursing workforce has probably contributed to the continued dominance of the medical profession. It has also made the development of integrated services fraught with difficulty. Nurses have made progress towards integrated nursing teams, but the value of teams which include only nurses has been questioned.[1]

The first contact service

In Britain, primary care is often seen as synonymous with general medical practice. Whilst in many areas this may appear to be the case, particularly for GPs who have worked in one practice for many years, the reality is very different. Primary care is the first contact service. It is that part of the health service which people consult when they first feel a need for help with aspects of their health. It is clear that there are a variety of settings in which this first contact can take place. There are also a variety of professionals providing a first contact service.

Nor are NHS settings the only places where first contacts happen. Within primary healthcare we might include occupational health services, school health services, alternative practitioners such as homeopaths, osteopaths and chiropractors, and parts of the voluntary sector. Within the NHS, first contacts may be with GPs, but they may also be with practice nurses, health visitors, midwives, accident and emergency departments (especially in inner cities) as well as NHS Direct and walk-in centres. It is important to remember that, in many settings, the first contact is normally made with a receptionist. It is often the receptionist who decides which professional the patient sees first.

An important feature of any 'first contact' service is that it is normally patient initiated. This is a vital distinction between primary care and other parts of the NHS.[2] GPs, for example, do not 'discharge' patients at the end of an episode of care. The person remains on the GP list, and may contact the doctor again at any time. Access to secondary care and hospital services is normally by referral from primary care.

The key skill required by all professional providers of a first contact service is that of assessment. They must be able to make a comprehensive assessment of the health care needs of the person who is asking for help. They must be generalists with a good knowledge of all aspects of health, and the ability to recognise deviations from the norm. This applies to mental as well as physical health. It also applies whatever the setting in which they are working. The professional label, doctor, nurse or whatever, is less important than the skills the professional has.

Developing primary mental healthcare

It has been known for decades that the majority of people with mental health problems are treated in primary care settings and are not referred for specialist care.[3] This is not because of the closure of large mental hospitals, nor the advent of care in the community. The increasing visibility to primary care staff of people with serious mental health problems is a separate issue from primary mental healthcare.

People with mental health problems in primary care are not a subspecies of people who are mad or crazy. They are an integral part of the primary care clientele. As well as their anxiety or depression, they may have heart disease, cancer, asthma or diabetes. They are not the 'worried well'.[4] 'Worried sick' might be a better description. Many of these people may be seriously disabled by their symptoms of depression or anxiety, but most do not require referral to specialist services. The priority for primary care should be to develop effective and responsive care for people with common mental health problems.

The focus of those who commission mental health services has been almost exclusively on severe mental illness (SMI). Clearly, care for these often highly vulnerable people has to be a priority for mental health services, but most of the definitions of SMI exclude most people with depression.[5] The focus on SMI has tended to distort primary care priorities and has left many GPs feeling that they are being asked to take on tasks which should, more appropriately, be done by the CMHT.

Practice nurses have also had concerns about this, especially when asked to provide depot neuroleptic medication for people with schizophrenia (*see* Chapter 6). Since most practice nurses are ill prepared for this task, the usual response has been to offer them training. It might be more appropriate to question whether they should be doing it at all. Arguably, they would be better occupied developing improved care for people with anxiety and depression.

The main roles for primary care teams in relation to people with SMI are to know who they are, and to provide proper physical healthcare. Once a register or care database is in place and the care of this group is being regularly and systematically monitored according to agreed care plans, then the team can turn its attention to the priority area for primary care – people with common mental health problems for whom there are few secondary care services.

Team approaches to mental healthcare

Depression is a chronic, relapsing illness. We have already seen that the traditional approach at primary care level is that contacts are initiated by the patient. Andrews points out that depression is an illness which reduces hope, motivation, treatment adherence and predisposes to suicide.[6] He suggests that the traditional reactive model of patient contact is inappropriate for such a condition and believes that chronic disease management models, such as those which exist for diabetes, might be more effective.

Gardner has described just such a model of care for depression, which she has developed over a number of years.[7] She points out that many practice nurses already have the necessary skills since they are experienced in chronic disease management. The skills are transferable. Her model 'general clinic' is conducted in collaboration with the GPs in the practice. She suggests that regular attendance at a clinic allowed the development of a therapeutic relationship between patient and nurse which empowers the patient and significantly improves outcome. The model has become known as the 'Orchard Model' and has been published in a toolkit designed to help primary care teams meet Standard 2 targets of the National Service Framework for Mental Health (Box 9.1).[8]

A practice team in Northamptonshire have looked in detail at the roles of all members in the care of patients with depression as part of an attempt to develop an integrated approach to mental healthcare.[9] This model acknowledges that all members of the team are likely to encounter such patients in the course of their day-to-day work and attempts to provide a framework within which all have a constructive part to play according to individual skills and training.

Box 9.1   The Orchard Model of care for people with depression

Aim: To improve the care of patients with depression in primary care.

Objectives:

- Identify patients with depression using a suitable assessment tool.
- Assess, plan and implement programme of care.
- Supervise patients taking medication to maximise treatment adherence.
- Monitor mood and suicide risk.
- Coordinate care in collaboration with other clinicians.

At the patient's first visit the nurse should:

- Administer appropriate questionnaire.
- Observe and record: mood, severity, duration, physical symptoms, social network and difficulties, view of self, suicidal thoughts.
- Assess needs, e.g. problem solving, information about medication, voluntary agencies/self-help groups, relaxation, general advice.
- Negotiate care plan.
- Refer back to prescribing GP in 2–4 weeks (earlier if suicidal ideas are present).

Thereafter:

- Routine follow-up approximately monthly. At each follow-up, assess: mood (re-administer questionnaire at appropriate intervals), treatment adherence, suicidal thinking, other symptoms.
- Refer back to GP if symptoms are worse, suicidal ideas present, drug side effects are intolerable, non-adherence to medication.

This model was pioneered at the Orchard Medical Practice, Ipswich. It is designed to be used by a practice nurse in collaboration with the patient's GP. It assumes that the patient is initially assessed by the GP and referred to the nurse for follow-up.

Table 9.1 is a modified version of this team's approach. They acknowledge that the process of achieving this type of integration is not painless. They have had to confront the tribalisms which exist within primary care teams. They suggest that one of the benefits has been that patients are receiving a more consistent approach to their care with all team members giving similar messages.

Moves to develop roles for a more specialist primary care mental health nurse have arisen in various parts of the country. In some cases this role is undertaken by a trained mental health nurse who may provide an assessment and treatment service for the primary care team. However, others believe that it is more appropriate that a primary care mental health nurse should in fact be a general nurse, with some extra training.[10] Primary care is a setting for generalists and the use of trained mental health nurses at this level may divert scarce specialist skills from the care of people with serious and enduring mental illness, as has happened in the past.[11]

Referral issues

Referral is often seen as a simple option of referral from a GP to specialist care. It is clear from Table 9.1 that within an integrated team there are opportunities for intra-team referral as well as referral outside. For example, there is likely to be referral between various members of the team and the practice counsellor. Many practices now have counsellors, but often they are far from integrated within the team. It may not be clear to all team members either what the counsellor does, or what kind of clients he or she will see. Box 9.2 may help to give some suitable criteria.

In the team depicted in Table 9.1 the CPN and the social worker are included. They will both accept referral from, and refer back to, other members of the team. This is helping to break down the barriers that have existed between primary and secondary care where CPNs and social workers are seen only as part of the community mental health team. Fairly clear guidelines on who to refer and when are required. Some teams may prefer to have more explicit protocols.

It is a requirement of the National Service Framework for Mental Health that protocols should be in place for common mental health problems and that these protocols should include criteria for referral to secondary care services. Developing these protocols needs to be a joint

Table 9.1 A team approach to depression care

	Practice nurse	Health visitor	CPN	Social worker	Counsellor	District nurse	GP
Client group	Everyone	Everyone, especially young mothers, families, carers, elderly people	Adults: (If over 65 to elderly team) (If under 16 to child and adolescent team)	Adults 18–65 Enduring/severe mental illness	Adults 16–65 Without psychotic symptoms	Elderly people, people discharged from hospital, carers	All
Assessment	Recognition Listening Facilitating Dealing with feelings Using scales	Use of EPDS, GDS As practice nurses	Scales, coping mechanisms, patients' views, trigger issues, support available	Risk assessment Assessment of needs: social, finance, housing, job, carers	Causes, options for intervention Hypothesis + coping mechanism + suicidality	Use of GDS As practice nurse	Suicidality Severity (scales) Patient view Support Social context Medication
Severity	Mild	Mild–moderate	Severe–moderate	Moderate–severe	Moderate–severe	Mild	All
When to refer/liaise	Suicidality Complex issues Failure to improve	Suicidality Complex issues Failure to improve	Neglect Safety issues Failure to improve	Patient wishes Complex social needs Family issues	Suicidality Complex issues Failure to improve	Suicidality Complex issues Failure to improve	Safety issues Failure to improve Patient wishes Family pressures
When to receive referrals	For advice and talking through leaflets – an educational role	Mothers of young children Help with postnatal depression Carers & isolated elderly	Moderate to severe especially at risk of self-harm Concurrent psychiatric illness	Advice on childcare, benefits, housing Moderate to severe risk esp. self-harm Concurrent psychiatric illness	Problems with personality development, especially people with relationship problems. stress, anxiety	People with other nursing needs impinging on their mood, e.g. physical disabilities, illness	Confirm diagnosis if unclear Multiaxial assessment Concern for other members of PHCT Medication

Adapted from Clark and Smart 1999 and the Northamptonshire GRiPP Project, Northamptonshire Health Authority 1998.[9,12]

exercise between primary and secondary care services. Though they might be initially developed at primary care trust/mental health trust level, all practice teams and CMHTs need to be aware of them. This must also include local co-ops and GP out-of-hours services as well as local crisis services.

Protocols are often confused with clinical guidelines, which may mean that they are wordy, detailed and far too long for any realistic expectation that anyone will read them, let alone implement them. Protocols may be better seen as patient 'care pathways' which simply explain what kind of care a patient should be receiving at any particular stage of their illness.

Referral to specialist clinical psychology services has caused particular problems for primary care. Waiting lists are often very long, sometimes up to nine months. Many primary care practitioners regard this as totally unacceptable, and may therefore not refer patients at all. There is some evidence that at least some long waiting lists may be the result of lack of clear referral criteria. Even though access to psychological therapies is acknowledged to be patchy and inadequate, what there is is possibly also being used inefficiently.[5]

Maintaining patients within primary care whilst they wait for these scarce therapies can be very stressful for members of the team. Strategies need to be in place to take some of the strain. Practice counsellors may be able to help. Alternatively there may be other local sources of therapy and/or support from the voluntary sector. Team members themselves will require support.

Box 9.2   Referring patients for counselling in primary care teams

Suitable clients will meet the following criteria but assessment is required in all cases:

1   their problems will affect their ability to cope with daily life, or the quality of their life and relationships
2   their problems will be causing current distress.

Indications of whether they will be able to use counselling effectively are:

1   being able to engage in conversation and willing to disclose personal information

2   having the capacity for reflection and some motivation for change
3   being willing and able to make a regular commitment to attend appointments.

The very fragile may well find counselling too challenging, as may those who have too much invested in remaining the same.

Clients amenable to counselling or psychotherapy in GP practices are likely to be those in the following categories:

- pathological bereavement
- coping with injury or illness
- depression – reactive, circumstantial
- developmental or life crises
- appropriate emotional, physical or sexual abuse issues
- family relationship issues
- general anxieties and phobias
- lack of direction, alienation, existential problems
- loss, e.g. relationship, employment, health, etc
- self-image and identity issues
- stress and trauma – pre and post event
- issues of sexuality.

Not all clients may be suitable for counselling or psychotherapy in GP practices. Specialist skills are required for the following:

- sexual dysfunction
- poor communication ability
- self-destructive behaviour, which, over time, has shown very little change, i.e. prolonged substance misuse, eating disorders
- moderate to severe mental illness/disorder
- severe challenging behaviour, i.e. aggression, violence, severe learning disabilities.

Supplied by Joan Foster, Association of Counsellors and Psychotherapists in Primary Care.

Clinical supervision

It is well recognised that clinical supervision should be an essential part of professional working. Counsellors are required by their organisations to have supervision on a regular basis. Nurses have been slow to recognise the need, particularly community nurses. Ross and Mackenzie (1996) have pointed out that as nurses, especially community nurses, develop increasingly autonomous roles, the need for effective clinical supervision becomes more and more apparent.[13] Not only is supervision a way of examining professional practice with the help of a skilled colleague, but it also provides support for sometimes isolated practitioners and aids reflective practice.

Conclusion

Nurses are likely to have increasing influence over the way primary care develops, especially as they become members of trust boards. Increasingly, it is nurses who are providing the 'first contact' service. This fact needs to be recognised at the highest levels in the NHS so that training needs will be met and appropriate support provided. Might it also be that when government ministers want answers to questions about primary health care, they will turn first to nurses and not to doctors? Nurses' perspectives are often wider, but they may be less confident in their knowledge.

It is also important that, as things change, mental health is recognised as being just as important to primary care as coronary heart disease, diabetes or asthma. We have an opportunity to look at new ways of providing, not just mental health care, but a completely integrated healthcare service. We need a system which does not simply pay lip service to ideas of holistic care, but genuinely seeks to address the range of mental, physical and social issues that affect the health of individuals, families and communities.

References

1   Elwyn G and Smail J (eds) (1999) *Integrated Teams in Primary Care* (Introduction). Radcliffe Medical Press, Oxford.

2   Armstrong E and Tylee AT (1999) Primary mental health care (Chapter 6). In: J Sims (ed.) *Primary Health Care Sciences.* Whurr Publishers, London.

3   Goldberg D and Huxley P (1982) *Mental Illness in the Community: the pathway to psychiatric care.* Tavistock, London.

4   Mann A (1992) Depression and anxiety in primary care: the epidemiological evidence (Chapter 1). In: R Jenkins, J Newton and R Young (eds) *The Prevention of Depression and Anxiety: the role of the primary care team.* HMSO, London.

5   Clinical Standards Advisory Group (CSAG) (1999) *Services for Patients with Depression.* Department of Health, London.

6   Andrews G (2001) Should depression be managed as a chronic disease? *BMJ.* **322**: 419–21.

7   Gardner S (1999) Practice nurses in mental health: a changing role? *J Primary Care Ment Health.* **2**: 11–12.

8   Armstrong E and Paton J (2001) *An Implementation Toolkit for Primary Care: The National Service Framework for Mental Health.* PriMHE, London.

9   Clark S and Smart D (1999) The integrated nursing team and primary care. *J Primary Care Ment Health.* **3**: 6–9.

10 Armstrong E (1995) *Mental Health Issues in Primary Care: a practical guide* (Chapter 9). Macmillan, London.

11 Goldberg D and Gournay K (1998) *The General Practitioner, the Psychiatrist and the Burden of Mental Health Care.* Maudsley discussion paper No. 1. Institute of Psychiatry, London.

12 Northamptonshire GRiPP (Getting Research into Practice and Purchasing) Project (1998) *Guidelines for the Recognition and Management of Depression in Primary Care.* Northamptonshire Health Authority.

13 Ross F and Mackenzie A (1996) New nursing roles in primary health care (Chapter 7). In: *Nursing in Primary Health Care: policy into practice.* Routledge, London.

Further reading

Blount A (ed.) (1998) *Integrated Primary Care. The Future of Medical and Mental Health Collaboration.* W Norton & Co, New York.

CHAPTER TEN

Promoting mental health and preventing mental illness

Elizabeth Armstrong

Introduction

In 1997, the Department of Health co-sponsored a London conference with the Royal Institute of Public Health and Hygiene and the World Health Organization. The theme of the conference was *Preventing Mental Illness: Mental Health Promotion in Primary Care*.

Worldwide, over 80% of people with mental health problems seek help from primary care providers.[1] In the UK, up to 90% of mental healthcare is provided solely by primary care. As Silva points out in the conference report, primary care is not confined to general medical practice. It encompasses workplaces, schools, health visiting services and a whole range of other sources of help. Thus there is huge challenge for primary care professionals to provide an environment which not only recognises and treats mental illness effectively and promptly, but also promotes the mental well-being of its clients.

Preventing mental illness

Not all mental illness is preventable. However, Newton suggested in the late eighties that we already had sufficient evidence to justify developing a preventive strategy for depression.[2] She has also suggested that three main features should characterise effective prevention-oriented services.[3]

- They should target the people known to be most at risk of developing a particular disorder.

- They should help people take control of their own lives without increasing their dependency on support services.
- They should make maximum use of voluntary, community and 'natural' caring networks (family and friends) and should not threaten resources for secondary care.

Preventive activities are often divided into three categories.

- *Primary prevention*: this is designed to prevent a disease happening at all. A useful example is immunisation.
- *Secondary prevention*: where early recognition and prompt effective treatment are designed to limit the severity and duration of a disease and, where possible, to prevent subsequent impairment. Cervical cytology, which aims to detect and treat pre-cancerous conditions of the cervix before serious disease develops, may be seen as an example of secondary prevention.
- *Tertiary prevention*: this has two aspects. Once illness and/or disability have occurred, tertiary prevention aims to help the individual maximise their remaining strengths and reduce any adverse effects on social functioning. Tertiary prevention may also be seen as attempts to reduce the likelihood of recurrence or relapse.

If these categories and Newton's principles are applied to depression, then:

- *Primary prevention* should aim to identify people who are at high risk of developing the illness and provide them with appropriate help to deal with their difficulties. The help provided should be empowering and should avoid creating dependency.
- *Secondary prevention* should aim to recognise and treat depression promptly with treatments which are known to be effective.
- *Tertiary prevention* should aim to continue treatment for as long as is appropriate to reduce the possibility of relapse; to teach patients skills which will help them avoid recurrence and to facilitate access to on-going support and care for those whose illness becomes chronic and associated with significant impairment.

Most of this can be done within the primary care setting. It is only those whose condition is life threatening (e.g. serious suicide risk); who fail to respond to primary care treatment or who have concurrent psychosis or drug or alcohol misuse who will require referral to secondary care services.

Secondary and tertiary prevention have been largely dealt with in Chapter 1. This chapter looks in more detail at opportunities for primary prevention.

Who is most at risk?

Chapter 1 has looked at the predisposing, precipitating, and maintaining factors for depressive illness. The risk factors can be summarised under the following headings.

- Bereavement and loss.
- Other major life changes such as moving house, leaving home to go to university or college, becoming a refugee.
- Relationship problems with spouse or partner, including sexual problems.
- Family difficulties (e.g. problems with adolescent children).
- Long-term caring responsibilities.
- Chronic, painful, life-threatening physical illness.
- Physical disability, particularly sight or hearing impairment.
- Social isolation.
- Work-related problems such as unemployment or fear of redundancy, bullying, harassment or discrimination.
- Other chronic social difficulties such as debt, deprivation, housing problems.
- Previous personal or family history of depression.

If asked, most people will admit to at least one, possibly two, risk factors. Furthermore, many people cope with incredible adversity without becoming depressed. In a well-known classic study, Brown and Harris described major life events as 'provoking agents' but believed these were not sufficient to cause depression on their own.[4] They considered that the effect of life events was not always additive. It does not necessarily follow that the greater the number of adverse events a person suffers, the more likely they are to become depressed. The actual adverse event may not be particularly important. It is the meaning that the event has for the individual which is significant. Brown and Harris also suggested that other factors, which they called vulnerability factors, were at work. They listed four factors which were significant in the women in their study:

- loss of own mother before the age of 11
- three or more children under 14 at home
- lack of a confiding relationship (perhaps with a partner, but not necessarily)
- lack of employment outside the home.

As well as these vulnerability factors, other influences include the individual's coping resources. Murray argues that those individuals with an 'internal locus of control' are less likely to become depressed.[5] This means that people who believe that they have some control over what happens to them are likely to cope with stressful events in more positive, energetic ways. High self-esteem is also linked to this sense of being able to influence events, rather than being controlled by them.

Murray also suggests that the higher rates of mental health problems found in deprived groups may be linked to poor coping mechanisms rather than deprivation *per se.* It appears that, for women at least, those who cope best with life stresses have a greater level of family support than those who become depressed and ill.

The nature of support

Some insight into the nature of effective social support is given by Barbee.[6] She noted four types of behaviour in the supporter, two of which worked and two of which did not. Positive behaviours included:

- problem solving – asking about stressful events and making suggestions about ways of coping
- emotional support – giving encouragement, affirming the person's ability, accepting the person's feelings as valid.

Unhelpful behaviours were:

- belittling the person's difficulties or substituting problems of their own
- avoiding the issue by pursuing their own agenda or trying to change the subject onto something else.

Brown has also looked at some criteria for effective support in a crisis:[7]

- the availability of a close confidant for the person 'at risk'
- active, on-going emotional support from the confidant
- the person providing support should avoid making negative comments about the person they are helping.

Practical primary prevention

It seems then, that a primary care preventive strategy needs to encompass at least two ways of helping and supporting those who might be at risk of developing a depressive illness. First, primary care teams will need a way of identifying people in the high-risk groups from amongst the practice population, or in individual nurse or health visitor caseloads. This will need to be linked to ways of helping these groups of people access the kinds of social support they need. Secondly, teams will need to be aware of appropriate means of providing support to people who are coping with life crises or transitions.

Effective Health Care (1997) suggested that long-term carers of highly dependent people were a high-risk group for whom there was evidence that preventive interventions may be helpful.[8] Other documents, including the National Service Framework for Mental Health, have suggested that practices should identify at-risk groups. For example, in Standard 6 a checklist for primary care teams is given. This is intended to help them help carers, specifically carers of people with mental health problems, but it is equally applicable to other carers. Teams should:

- identify those of their patients who are carers, and patients who have a carer
- check the physical and emotional health of carers opportunistically, but at least once a year
- ensure that all carers know that they can ask social services for an assessment of their own needs
- always ask patients who have carers whether health information may be shared with their carer
- know about local carers' support groups and centres in their area and tell carers about them.

Identification of carers may not be as simple as it sounds. In theory, practice computers ought to be the source of most of this kind of information.

However, the information may not be recorded in an accessible way, if indeed it is recorded at all. Sources other than the practice computer will need to be consulted. These might include the community mental health team (for carers of people with mental health problems), community mental health teams for the elderly and district nurses (for carers of people with dementia), health visitors and community learning disabilities teams (for families with disabled children and carers of people with learning disabilities). Social services may also have some information, particularly about young carers, who may be an especially disadvantaged group.

Effective Health Care (1997) suggests that useful ways of providing preventive help to carers may include group sessions combined with training in assertiveness and coping skills.[8] This bulletin also suggested that other key groups whose needs should be targeted include:

- children who are:
  - living in poverty
  - exhibiting behavioural difficulties
  - experiencing parental separation and divorce
  - living in families experiencing bereavement.

- adults who are:
  - undergoing divorce or separation
  - unemployed
  - at risk of depression in pregnancy
  - experiencing bereavement.

In all of these instances, it would seem to be important that before offering support from their own resources the primary care team should ascertain what other sources of support people have. They should also, where possible, point people to appropriate sources of help within the community such as voluntary agencies and self-help groups. This presupposes that the primary care team itself has access to this information. A local directory, wall chart or on-line system showing available services and their contact details will be useful.

'Signposting' is not, nor should it be, referral in the medical sense. Iliffe and colleagues have described the process as 'networking'.[9] The primary care team enters and becomes part of the local network of social services, voluntary organisations, religious organisations and other bodies. Thus the team gets to know local agencies and to have confidence in them and the services they provide. The Amalthea Project in Avon has demonstrated that facilitated contact with voluntary agencies improved the outcome for patients in several ways.[10] These included reduced mental health scores, finding it easier to carry out everyday activities and more positive feelings about quality of life. Signposting may also be an essential component of providing support to people experiencing life crises.

In the main, there are two ways of dealing with stressful situations – either change the situation or, if the situation cannot be changed, then learn ways of coping with it. For the professional, therefore, the main ways of supporting people in some form of crisis may be either problem solving or helping people learn coping strategies. Some people will already have some methods of coping. These can be reinforced if appropriate and not damaging. Inappropriate coping strategies such as heavy drinking may need to be discouraged and better ones substituted. The Strategies for Living Project from the Mental Health Foundation is providing a mass of information about the things people with mental health problems find useful.

Promoting mental health

Practice teams then, require the means to identify and target help towards groups in the practice population who might be considered to be at high risk of developing mental health problems, especially depression. This will include ways of helping those experiencing life crises. Both of these measures may be seen as health promoting as well as preventive, but there are some other aspects of promoting mental health which any team may wish to consider.

Some of these are listed in Standard 1 of the National Service Framework and may already be in place. For example, many health visitors provide emotional support for mothers and may facilitate access to sources of support within the community such as groups run by the National Childbirth Trust. Some health visitors have set up their own groups for mothers who find it difficult to cope, sometimes in collaboration with local community mental health teams.[11] Papworth and Taylor describe a practice-based project in Northumbria in which efforts were made towards helping vulnerable mothers strengthen the factors which would make psychological distress less likely.[12] These include such things as boosting social support, improving self-esteem and positive coping abilities and facilitating access to existing resources such as child-care and family support schemes. This project was a collaboration between a health visitor and a clinical psychologist.

Domestic violence, in which women are the most frequent victims, was also a concern of the National Service Framework. Such violence may come to the attention of primary care team members, but a study by Frost suggested that, for health visitors at least, there was a huge need for training in this area.[13] She also found that many health visitors felt vulnerable in situations where clients were experiencing violence from a partner. The quality of guidance on personal safety and support for health visitors from their employers was felt to be variable and patchy. It is likely that the situation is similar across practice teams.

The mental health aware practice

It has been suggested elsewhere that the practice which wants to promote the mental well-being of its patients needs to do more than detect and treat illness early.[14] The benefits of attention to the whole atmosphere in which care is delivered will be apparent not only in a less stressed work-force, but also in less anxiety on the part of patients and probably less aggressive behaviour too. It has been highlighted elsewhere in this book that the first patient contact in any practice setting is normally with the receptionists. Well-trained and supported receptionists will be able to greet patients sensitively and help them find the right person in the team to address their problems.

There are still many practices working in premises which are less than ideal, with consulting rooms and clinics at the top of steep staircases, cramped and dark waiting rooms and dingy corridors. Confidentiality at the reception desk can be a problem if waiting room chairs are too close. A great deal can be done with a creative use of plants, soft furnishings, screens and pictures to make practice premises more welcoming and reception areas more private. Patient groups may be able to help with some of this.

Rogers and colleagues, in a study for the Health Education Authority, looked at lay views of mental health and mental ill health.[15] They found that many people did not regard their GP as an appropriate person to confide in about emotional difficulties. It may be that nurses are seen as more approachable – there is some evidence from the nursing literature that this may be so – but this study found that most people in distress would prefer to talk with a friend or family member. The availability of patient information such as leaflets and posters about depression along-side other health information may help to create an atmosphere of accep-tance and encourage people who need help to ask for it.

All practice staff should be appropriately trained to be aware of and sen-sitive to the needs of the particular area in which they work, including awareness of local cultural differences and the needs of minority ethnic groups in their localities (*see* Chapter 8). Where feasible, one member of staff might wish to take on the responsibility of building links with local ethnic community leaders. All practice staff, administrative as well as pro-fessional, should also have some understanding of the needs of people with mental illness to avoid the pervasive discrimination which may lead to their health needs being ignored.

Dealing with aggression

Aggressive behaviour on the part of some patients has become an impor-tant issue for many practices especially, but not exclusively, those in inner-city areas. It is important that practice staff, particularly the recep-tion staff who man the 'front desk', have training in how to deal with aggressive patients and, where possible, to prevent or diffuse violence. Braithwaite believes that the most common reaction to aggressive or vio-lent behaviour is to freeze.[16] Freezing occurs because the recipient is shocked or afraid. He suggests that freezing needs to be countered. Action should replace inaction. The recipient of the aggression needs to be able to either act to calm the situation, or to flee if physical danger seems immi-nent. This takes practice.

Aggressive behaviour may be calmed using a six-stage plan.

1   Stay calm: take a deep breath and exhale slowly before speaking.
2   Show concern: assume that there is a reason for the behaviour.
3   Acknowledge the aggression – say something like 'I can see that you're angry'.
4   Try to diffuse the situation, for example by requesting that the beha-viour stops. Say something like 'Please stop shouting and I'll see if I can help you'.

5 Identify the cause and try to find a solution. This should be possible, if the aggressor calms down.
6 Agree with the aggressor a different way of behaving in future.

(Adapted from Braithwaite 1992.[16])

If, at any time, the aggression does not appear to be lessening, or is getting worse, get help or leave the situation. Staff need to be trained not to put themselves in physical danger.

Staff mental health

Staff who are under stress or depressed themselves are unlikely to be able to give of their best to their patients and clients. Traditionally, primary care has lagged seriously behind other parts of the health service in providing support for staff. Access to occupational health services is still inadequate in many areas. Clinical supervision is only slowly becoming available for practice nurses. Even health visitors working with mothers with postnatal depression may find their access to clinical supervision is patchy and inconsistent.

There has been increasing attention in recent years to the level of stress-related disorders in doctors. Evidence is accumulating that disorders such as depression may be equally prevalent in nurses. Brandon reports on a survey of nurses' experiences of being treated for depression.[17] More than half of those questioned cited work as the main cause of their illness. Brandon believes that many of the nurses in the survey left their jobs as a result of unhelpful attitudes from their managers or employers, in some cases GPs.

There is also evidence that female nurses in particular are at increased risk of suicide. The reasons for this are unclear, but Hawton and Vislisel speculate that a sense of autonomy appears to be associated with reduced stress.[18] In addition, those nurses who are more assertive appear to have lower depression scores. Access to means may be a less important risk factor for suicide in female nurses than it is, for example, in doctors, vets and farmers.

It is worrying that the great attention given to stress in doctors detracts from work needed to improve working lives and support for all healthcare professionals. Nurses can be forgiven sometimes for believing they are the invisible part of the workforce. Perhaps the above research should encourage more nurses to be more assertive about the problems they face and demand better support from their employers.

Conclusion

Friedli believes that mental health promotion is mainly about the way individuals, families, organisations and communities feel, what it is that influences these feelings and the effect this has on health and well-being.[19] She makes the point, too, that although prevention, treatment and cure are important, none of these things do much to influence the way we feel.

The ability of health professionals to promote mental health is necessarily limited. So many things impinge on mental well-being, a large proportion of which are not under the direct influence of doctors and nurses. But this is not a reason for doing nothing. Friedli suggests that mental health promotion works at three levels:

- strengthening individuals, for example by interventions which enhance self-esteem and coping skills
- strengthening communities, for example by building health and social services that support mental health
- reducing the structural barriers to mental health, for example by initiatives which reduce discrimination and inequality.

It is clear from this that at all three levels there are things that primary care professionals, teams and organisations can do to provide a mental health promoting service.

References

1 Silva JAC (1998) World Health Organization perspectives and prevention of mental illness and mental health promotion in primary care (Chapter 2). In: R Jenkins and TB Ustun (eds) *Preventing Mental Illness. Mental Health Promotion in Primary Care.* John Wiley and Sons Ltd, Chichester.

2 Newton J (1989) *Preventing Mental Illness.* Routledge, London.

3 Newton J (1992) Crisis support: utilising resources. In: R Jenkins, J Newton and R Young (eds) *The Prevention of Depression and Anxiety: the role of the primary care team.* HMSO, London.

4 Brown GW and Harris TO (1978) *The Social Origins of Depression.* Tavistock, London.

5 Murray J (1995) *The Prevention of Anxiety and Depression in Vulnerable Groups.* Gaskell, London.

6 Barbee AP (1990) Interactive coping: the cheering up process in close relationships. In: S Duck (ed.) *Personal Relationships and Social Support.* Sage Publications, London.

7 Brown GW (1992) Life events and social support: possibilities for primary prevention. In: R Jenkins, J Newton and R Young (eds) *The Prevention of Depression and Anxiety: the role of the primary care team.* HMSO, London.

8 Effective Health Care (1997) Mental health promotion in high-risk groups. *Effective Health Care Bulletin.* **3**(3) NHS Centre for Reviews and Dissemination, University of York.

9 Iliffe S, Patterson L and Gould MM (1998) *Health Care for Older People* (Chapter 5). BMJ Books, London.

10 Grant C, Goodenough T, Harvey I *et al.* (2000) A randomised controlled trial and economic evaluation of a referrals facilitator between primary care and the voluntary sector. *BMJ.* **320**: 419–23.

11 Foyster L (1995) Supporting mothers: an interdisciplinary approach. *Health Visitor.* **68**(4): 151–2.

12 Papworth M and Taylor K (2000) Psychological difficulties: a GP practice approach. *Community Pract.* **73**(1): 439–41.

13 Frost M (1997) Health visitors' perceptions of domestic violence. *Health Visitor.* **70**(7): 258–9.

14 Armstrong E (1995) *Mental Health Issues in Primary Care: a practical guide* (Chapter 8). Macmillan, London.

15 Rogers A, Pilgrim D and Latham M (1996) *Understanding and Promoting Mental Health.* Health Education Authority, London.

16 Braithwaite R (1992) *Violence: understanding, intervention and prevention* (Chapter 13). Radcliffe Medical Press, Oxford.

17 Brandon D (2001) Wounded healers. *Open Mind.* **108**: 10–11.

18 Hawton K and Vislisel L (1999) Suicide in nurses. *Suicide Life Threat Behav.* **29**(1): 86–95.

19 Friedli L (2000) Mental health promotion: how do you feel? *J Primary Care Ment Health.* **4**(2): 30–2.

Further reading

Strategies for Living: newsletter from the Mental Health Foundation (*see* Appendix).

Tylee A, Kendrick T and Freeling P (1996) *The Prevention of Mental Illness in Primary Care*. Cambridge University Press, Cambridge.

CHAPTER ELEVEN

Conclusion: final thoughts

Elizabeth Armstrong

We began this book with a brief look at the National Service Framework for Mental Health and saw that the framework is intended to improve the quality of mental healthcare for all patients, not just those who are receiving their care from specialist services. The framework did acknowledge that primary care nurses have a role in this, but there were no primary care nurses on the external reference group that compiled it so references to nurses and nursing were sparse, unimaginative and not particularly well informed.

Moreover, the framework was couched in language more commonly associated with specialist services than with primary care. For example, even in Standard 2 which was primarily about primary care, patients were referred to as 'service users'. This is a term not widely used in primary care, except perhaps to refer to people who are being treated by specialist psychiatric services. Some confusion about this standard is therefore hardly surprising.

A careful reading reveals that, in fact, this standard is about people with common mental health problems who are, as the framework makes clear, only rarely referred to specialists. In other words, despite its confusing language, this standard is about primary care and the primary care clientele.

Primary care mental health is not psychiatry. In the main, people attending their GP surgery neither want nor need referral to a psychiatric specialist. In most instances, a psychiatric label may be less than helpful. A proportion of people with severe depression or anxiety will acquire a formal diagnosis and receive medication as well as other therapies. Very often there will be no formal diagnosis, possibly because of the stigma which still attaches to any mental illness and possibly because patients are reluctant to have such diagnoses on their national insurance certificates.

But people with mild to moderate symptoms still need help. It has been an aim of this book to provide some ways in which effective help can be given in primary care settings, sometimes by nurses working in collaboration with GPs, sometimes working in collaboration with other professionals such as counsellors or community mental health nurses. The clear theme is that this is an area of care in which general nurses not only should be involved, but are involved whether they recognise it or not.

It should no longer be professionally acceptable to say that, as a general nurse, it is not your job to work with people with mental health problems. As has been highlighted elsewhere, people with mental health problems are not a sub-species of crazy or mad individuals. They are the same people the practice nurse is seeing for their travel immunisations, diabetic checks, cervical smears and so on. They are the same mother the health visitor is visiting with a new baby, a toddler needing a developmental check or a child about to start school. They are the same patient the district nurse is seeing with a terminal illness or the person caring for a disabled relative. They are the bread and butter of primary care.

Mental health is part of healthcare, not an optional extra. The problem is that for many general nurses working in primary care settings, mental health and illness did not feature much in their initial training and, where it did, it was likely to have been confined to a short spell on a psychiatric ward in hospital. Poor preparation for the realities of the community! It is well documented that the average age of the community nursing workforce tends to be older than its hospital counterpart. Whilst maturity is an essential requisite for community nursing, it may mean that initial training was a long time ago and, until fairly recently, there have been few opportunities for primary care nurses to update their mental health knowledge.

Nevertheless, there are many who have found the means and there are practice nurses involved in innovative projects to improve mental health care in their practices. Health visitors are now the main source of help for mothers with postnatal depression, but training is not always available, and post-training support may be patchy. Patients on the traditional district nurse caseload are often at high risk of developing mental health problems but there may be little awareness amongst these nurses, or their managers, that training is required in order to effectively meet patient need. Training opportunities are only going to improve if nurses themselves demand that they do.

A second aim of this book has been to encourage nurses to play their full part at all levels in primary care, both as skilled practitioners caring directly for patients, and also as professionals with an interest in developing the service as a whole. Primary care, as the first contact service, is already largely delivered by nurses. In the future, more and more of it will be delivered by nurses. But will nurses be content to deliver a service that was good enough for the last century, or will they want to take a lead in developing a service for the 21st?

The concept of primary care mental health is still relatively new. The way is open for it to be shaped in a way which much better meets the needs of the customers, all the customers from whichever social or cultural group they come. Nurses, as members of PCG and PCT boards, have unprecedented opportunities to influence the way primary care develops, but they will need to be assertive and brave enough to speak up for the values they believe in.

There is a unique opportunity to bring mental healthcare into the main stream. There is allegedly government money attached to the implementation of the National Service Framework, and mental health is one of the three main priorities. But mental health is not as glamorous or as appealing to the media as heart disease or cancer. It can easily get overlooked and funds can be, and are, diverted into what seem like more pressing issues. If there is a choice of funding a course on coronary heart disease or one on depression, there will be no prizes for guessing which wins!

Primary care mental health needs champions. Some of these could be nurses.

Appendix: Resources

Questionnaires and screening tools

Hospital Anxiety and Depression Scale (HADS)

This scale is copyright. It may be purchased in bulk, together with information on its use, from:

NFER-Nelson Publishing Company Limited
Darville House
2 Oxford Road East
Windsor
Berks SL4 1BU

The Goldberg General Health Questionnaire is available from the same source.

Edinburgh Postnatal Depression Scale (EPDS)

This scale is available from a variety of sources. It may be copied with appropriate acknowledgements. For detailed information on its use, see Cox J and Holden J (1994) *Perinatal Psychiatry: use and misuse of the Edinburgh Postnatal Depression Scale.* Gaskell, London.

The Beck Depression Inventory is mainly used by specialists. Copies may be available from your local CMHT. Alternatively, copies are available from the Royal College of Psychiatrists (*see* p. 148).

Sources of patient information

MIND
Granta House
15–19 Broadway
Stratford
London E15 4BQ

Tel: 020 8519 2122 (for publications: ext 219)
www.mind.org.uk

National Schizophrenia Fellowship
28 Castle Street
Kingston-on-Thames
Surrey KT1 1SS

Advice service: (Monday to Friday 10 am to 3 pm) 020 8974 6814
www.nsf.org.uk

Depression Alliance
35 Westminster Bridge Road
London SE1 7JB

Tel: 020 7633 0557
Fax: 020 7633 0559
www.depressionalliance.org.uk

Association for Postnatal Illness
25 Jerdan Place
London SW6 1BE

Tel: 020 7386 0868

Mental Health Foundation
20–21 Cornwall Street
London NW1 4QL

Tel: 020 7535 7400
Fax: 020 7535 7474
www.mentalhealth.org.uk

Eating Disorders Association
First Floor, Wensum House
103 Prince of Wales Road
Norwich NR1 1DW

Helplines: 01603 621414 (9 am to 6.30 pm weekdays)
Youthline: 01603 765050 (4 pm to 6 pm weekdays)
www.edauk.com

Manic Depression Fellowship
8–10 High Street
Kingston-on-Thames
Surrey KT1 1EY

Tel: 020 8974 6550
www.mdf.org.uk

SANE
199–205 Old Marylebone Road
London NW1 5QP

SANELINE: (2 pm to midnight every day) 08456 678000 (outside London)
020 7724 8000 (in London)

Alzheimer's Disease Society
Gordon House
10 Greencoat Place
London SW1P 1PH

Tel: 020 7306 0606

Young Minds Trust
22a Boston Place
London NW1 6ER

Tel: 020 7336 8445

Talking Life (for audio tapes on a variety of mental health-related topics)
Wendy Lloyd Audio Productions
1a Grosvenor Road
Hoylake
Wirral CH47 3BS

Tel: 0151 632 0662
www.talkinglife.co.uk

Videos for Patients
PO Box 22547
London W8 7GW

Tel: 020 7727 2690
Fax: 020 7727 2673
www.videosforpatients.co.uk

Samaritans National Helpline: 08457 909090
www.samaritans.org.uk

Sources of professional information

PriMHE
The Old Stables
2a Laurel Avenue
Twickenham TW1 4JA

Tel: 020 8891 6593
www.primhe.org.uk

Royal College of Psychiatrists
17 Belgrave Square
London SW1

Tel: 020 7235 2351
www.rcpsych.org.uk

Sainsbury Centre for Mental Health
134–138 Borough High Street
London SE1 1LB

Tel: 020 7403 8790
www.scmh.org.uk

Counselling in Primary Care Trust
Suite 3a
Majestic House
High Street
Staines TW18 4DG

Tel: 01784 441782
Fax: 01784 442601
www.cpct.co.uk

Association of Counsellors and Psychotherapists in Primary Care
95 Hewarts Lane
Bognor Regis
West Sussex PO21 3DJ

Tel: 01243 268322
Fax: 01243 268433
Email: cpc@cpct.co.uk

WHO Guide to Mental Health in Primary Care: www.whoguidemhpcuk.org

Sources of training in mental health for primary care

Depression Care Training Centre Limited
University College, Northampton
Thornby 1, Park Campus
Boughton Green Road
Northampton NN2 7AL

Tel: 01604 735500 ext 2640
Fax: 01604 712425
www.depressioncaretraining.org
Email: liz.armstrong@northampton.ac.uk

Index